BECOMING GODS

MEDICAL ANTHROPOLOGY: HEALTH, INEQUALITY, AND SOCIAL JUSTICE

Series editor: Lenore Manderson

Books in the Medical Anthropology series are concerned with social patterns of and social responses to ill health, disease, and suffering, and how social exclusion and social justice shape health and healing outcomes. The series is designed to reflect the diversity of contemporary medical anthropological research and writing, and will offer scholars a forum to publish work that showcases the theoretical sophistication, methodological soundness, and ethnographic richness of the field.

Books in the series may include studies on the organization and movement of peoples, technologies, and treatments, how inequalities pattern access to these, and how individuals, communities and states respond to various assaults on wellbeing, including from illness, disaster, and violence.

For a list of all the titles in the series, please see the last page of the book.

BECOMING GODS

Medical Training in Mexican Hospitals

VANIA SMITH-OKA

RUTGERS UNIVERSITY PRESS
New Brunswick, Camden, and Newark, New Jersey, and London

Library of Congress Cataloging-in-Publication Data
Names: Smith-Oka, Vania, 1975– author.
Title: Becoming gods : medical training in Mexican hospitals / Vania Smith-Oka.
Description: New Brunswick, New Jersey : Rutgers University Press, [2021] |
     Series: Medical anthropology | Includes bibliographical references and index.
Identifiers: LCCN 2020043991 | ISBN 9781978819665 (hardcover) |
     ISBN 9781978819658 (paperback) | ISBN 9781978819672 (epub) |
     ISBN 9781978819689 (mobi) | ISBN 9781978819696 (pdf)
Subjects: LCSH: Interns (Medicine)—Mexico—Puebla de Zaragoza. | Medical
     education—Social aspects—Mexico—Puebla de Zaragoza. | Teaching
     hospitals—Mexico—Puebla de Zaragoza. | Medical anthropology—
     Mexico—Puebla de Zaragoza.
Classification: LCC R840 .S65 2021 | DDC 610.71/55097248—dc23
LC record available at https://lccn.loc.gov/2020043991

A British Cataloging-in-Publication record for this book is available from the
British Library.

♾ The paper used in this publication meets the requirements of the American
National Standard for Information Sciences—Permanence of Paper for Printed
Library Materials, ANSI Z39.48-1992.

www.rutgersuniversitypress.org

Manufactured in the United States of America

For my parents, Pauline and Christopher

CONTENTS

ILLUSTRATIONS

FIGURES

TABLES

FOREWORD

LENORE MANDERSON

Medical Anthropology: Health, Inequality and Social Justice aims to capture the diversity of contemporary medical anthropological research and writing. The beauty of ethnography is its capacity, through storytelling, to make sense of suffering as a social experience and to set it in context. Central to our focus in this series, therefore, is the way in which social structures, political-economic systems, and ideologies shape the likelihood and impact of infections, injuries, bodily ruptures and disease, chronic conditions and disability, treatment and care, social repair, and death.

Health and illness are social facts; the circumstances of the maintenance and loss of health are always and everywhere shaped by structural, local, and global relations. Social formations and relations, culture, economy, and political organization as much as ecology shape the variance of illness, disability, and disadvantage. The authors of the monographs in this series are concerned centrally with health and illness, healing practices, and access to care, but in each case they highlight the importance of such differences in context as expressed and experienced at individual, household, and wider levels: health risks and outcomes of social structure and household economy, for instance, health systems factors, and national and global politics and economics all shape people's lives. In their accounts of health, inequality, and social justice, the authors move across social circumstances, health conditions, and geography, and their intersections and interactions, to demonstrate how individuals, communities, and states manage assaults on people's health and well-being.

As medical anthropologists have long illustrated, the relationships of social context and health status are complex. In addressing these questions, the authors in this series showcase the theoretical sophistication, methodological rigor, and empirical richness of the field, while expanding a map of illness and social and institutional life to illustrate the effects of material conditions and social meanings in troubling and surprising ways. The books reflect medical anthropology as a constantly changing field of scholarship, drawing on research diversely in residential and virtual communities, in clinics and laboratories, and in emergency care and public health settings with service providers, individual healers, and households, with social bodies, human bodies, and biologies. Although medical anthropology once concentrated on systems of healing, particular diseases, and embodied experiences, today the field has expanded to include environmental disaster, war, science, technology, faith, gender-based violence, and forced migration. Curiosity about the body and its vicissitudes remains pivotal to our work, but our concerns are with the location of bodies in social life and with how social structures, temporal imperatives, and shifting exigencies shape life courses. This dynamic field reflects an ethics of the discipline to address these pressing issues of our time.

Globalization has contributed to and adds to the complexity of influences on health outcomes; it (re)produces social and economic relations that institutionalize poverty, unequal conditions of everyday life and work, and environments in which diseases increase or subside. Globalization has patterned the movement and relations of peoples, technologies, and knowledge, programs, and treatments; it shapes differences in health experience and outcomes across space; it informs and amplifies inequalities at both individual and country levels. Global forces and local inequalities compound and constantly weigh on individuals, impacting their physical and mental health, and their households and communities. At the same time, as the subtitle of this series indicates, we are concerned with questions of social exclusion and inclusion, social justice and repair, again both globally and in local settings. The books will challenge readers to reflect not only on sickness and suffering, deficit and despair, but also on resistance and restitution—on how people respond to injustices and evade the fault lines that might seem to predetermine life outcomes. The aim is to widen the frame within which we conceptualize embodiment and suffering.

The capacity to heal is revered everywhere, yet anthropology's interest in the acquisition of the knowledge, skills, techniques, and arts of healing has been primarily for spiritual healers, including the revelation of their vocation, their initiation and induction, and their herbs and fetishes, appurtenances, and possessions. In these conventionally low-income settings, training takes place through apprenticeship to other experienced healers, midwives, shamans, and herbalists, in their own homes and in sacred dedicated spaces.

We have attended far less to the training of practitioners from any modality—Ayurveda, Traditional Chinese Medicine, Unani medicine, or cosmopolitan biomedicine—in professionalized, institutional settings. Yet the largest number of healers worldwide are biomedical doctors, nurses, and allied health professionals, trained in Western-style university medical schools and hospitals. In *Becoming Gods: Medical Training in Mexican Hospitals,* Vania Smith-Oka takes us, as readers, to two hospitals in the city of Puebla, southeast of Mexico City, and shows us how senior students of medicine become doctors in this setting.

Doctors become "gods" because they hold life and death in their hands. But the capacity to do this is learned. In Mexico, in their fifth year of training, medical students become hospital interns apprenticed to junior graduate doctors or residents. Sometimes also in the presence of established clinicians and specialists they study the art of clinical practice, and so earn the right to enter a pantheon. In the total institution of the hospital, on the lowest rungs of an insistent hierarchy, these trainees learn the codes of practice, the technologies and procedures, and the ideologies, attitudes, and values of being a doctor and becoming gods. Armed with the accoutrements of their practice—surgical scrubs, white coats, stethoscopes, and clipboards—they work impossibly long hours. They are sustained by the adrenaline of the excitement of medical emergencies and precarious lives and the challenges of acquiring the embodied hands-on skills of clinical assessment and care. At the same time, they are frustrated and demoralized by hospital bureaucracies and petty record keeping, run-down buildings, staff shortages, stock outages of drugs and other supplies, patient resistance, and the culpability and bullying of those who they are supposed to emulate.

In the shadows of Mexico's political and economic instability, drug violence, and structural vulnerability, trainees learn the habitus of being doctors as these are shaped by structural and social factors, and as complicated within the hospitals by medical hierarchies, race, ethnicity, class, and gender. The latter stands out. Smith-Oka's accounts of intentional, malicious violence against women are shocking: the harassment and victimization of female interns, the everyday sexism, and the physical, verbal, and emotional abuse of and unjustified obstetric interventions on female patients. The promised rewards of being a doctor allow trainees to stay the distance, as they constantly witness injustice, share in its perpetration, and rile against it.

Becoming Gods is provocative and deeply troubling. In Mexico—but also likely worldwide—we train young people to be doctors and to practice medicine without humility, care, or grace for people who are vulnerable and frightened, often desperately ill, and most likely too poor and too powerless to resist. Smith-Oka unfolds this account of doctor-making through rich ethnography and history, sensitivity and insight, and we are left to reflect on the small miracle: that a system of education and training that is often brutal and callous can produce so many doctors who are, despite it, deeply committed to the ethics of care.

BECOMING GODS

INTRODUCTION
Medicine as an (Extra)Ordinary Social Commitment

Those who are occupied in the restoration of health to others, by the joint exertion of skill and humanity, are above all the great of the earth. They even partake of divinity, since to preserve and renew is almost as noble as to create. —Voltaire

[Patients] arrive here, and they see people wearing a white coat, and, I don't know, they entrust their lives to them. It's also cool they think that we are better than them, when in reality all we do is examine them and we know what medications or procedures are needed.... I believe [doctors] are like an extension of God's hand. —Ricardo, intern at Hospital Piedad

"We have a bus accident coming in; a couple dozen patients will be arriving in one hour." The phone call came in at 1:30 A.M., reminding the interns doing an overnight shift at Hospital Piedad in the city of Puebla, Mexico that their time belonged to the hospital. They had just settled down on the two bunk beds in the hospital residence for what seemed like an uneventful night when the message about the accident was sent from the emergency room. A trailer on an eighteen-wheeler truck had come apart, veering across the midnight highway, and the bus struck it frontally. The bus driver was crushed in the wreckage—killed on impact. No one knew the extent of the passengers' injuries.

Hoping to sleep for a while before the patients arrived, the interns curled up on bunks, two to a bed, stethoscopes and white coats hanging from bedposts. Megan (my research assistant) and I shared a lower bunk, our white coats over us as we tried to sleep. Less than two hours later we were buzzed awake by phone calls. "Doctors, come to the ER now!"

Grabbing their stethoscopes, glasses, and clipboards, the interns pulled their white coats over their sleep-rumpled scrubs and dashed along the dark hospital passages toward the brightly lit emergency room (ER).[1] The scrubs, white coats, clipboards, and able hands transformed them from sleep-deprived interns to competent superheroes and gods in the medical ward. I followed them, notebook and pen in hand, my arms trembling from the adrenaline rush. This event, though extraordinary to the victims of the accident and to the anthropologist, was ordinary for the medical personnel. It was one of a thousand harried learning moments, where the extraordinary nature of the tragedy was transformed into ordinary and normative.

It was 3:30 A.M. The air was tense, but under control. The clinicians had to work quickly. Gabriel, a very competent and thoughtful intern, was in triage with a young female patient. Israel and Diego filled out paperwork at the nurses' station.[2] They were joined by Sebastián and Julieta. César, his hair in disarray, tensely clicked his pen as he strode by with a form in his hand. I hovered by them, feeling increasingly useless. I turned to Julieta and offered my help; she said, "I'll tell you in a minute how to fill out the [forms]." She then handed me an intake form and told me I could help her by writing down the patient's name, age, family history, medical history, their symptoms, and reason for being here. She was familiar with this process, quickly noting the main details about the accident: "Frontal crash, against a trailer that separated from the truck carrying it," and details about the patient's impact during the crash—whether it was frontal or lateral and what parts of the bus they struck. In contrast to the practiced flow of her narrative, mine was choppy as I awkwardly wrote down patients' answers to questions, uncertain of what was medically important to include and what was not.

Because this was a highway accident, it fell under the jurisdiction of the *Ministerio Público,* the national jurisprudence and prosecutorial ministry. In addition to all the paperwork the interns were expected to fill out for each patient, they also had to complete Ministerio forms reporting the details of the accident, which would be used for insurance purposes. After they filled out the many forms, the doctor on call signed each one. Some interns whose patients had already been released took advantage to catch a few minutes of sleep back at the residence, to the dismay of those who were still waiting for results from X-rays and other medical tests. At 7:00 A.M., as the last patient was rolled away by orderlies, the interns staggered back to the residence to shower and begin their day with patients, examinations, and paperwork.

For the interns, who are students in their fifth year of medical training, this was what I term an extraordinary, ordinary night. It was ordinary because every day at the hospital they had to deal with patients, doctors, paperwork, and technology, and to do so with little to no sleep. The bulk of their training came from the ordinary minutiae of medical care. The practice of such minutiae slowly transformed them from hesitant neophyte "doctors," who barely knew how to do basic procedures such as suturing or intake forms, into experienced physicians who could confidently navigate hospital spaces and patient bodies. But the night was also extraordinary. Bus accidents were not a regular part of the interns' routine or even of their training, and they had to rapidly figure out what they needed to do and do it well. The extraordinary occurred rarely, but the halls of medicine are awash with such stories. These events form the basis of prevailing fears and anxiety, essentially shaping how medicine is learned. And yet it is in the ordinary where medical transformation is most profound and where its effect can be most impactful on patient lives. Interns' responses to both the extraordinary and the ordinary become yardsticks to gauge their commitment to medicine.

In this book, I employ this ordinary–extraordinary heuristic to explain how medical knowledge, skills, and attitudes are transmitted within hospital spaces, how sometimes things that should be ordinary (like vaginal birth) become extraordinary, and how some practices that should be extraordinary (like bullying or obstetric violence) become ordinary. I explore how medical students in Mexico transform into fledgling physicians over their year-long internship, acquiring a medical self. Within this dynamic setting, interns develop a medical self in the ordinary spaces and experiences—navigating a medical ward, sleeping few hours, learning to speak with patients from different backgrounds, as well as with doctors, nurses, and colleagues, presenting cases, embodying medical and social values, and handling new equipment—as well as in the extraordinary—learning to manage stress when a patient goes into cardiac arrest, identifying themselves with the stories of struggling doctors elsewhere, figuring out whether to empathize or not with a patient who arrives with a stillbirth pregnancy, or treating bus accident patients. I draw from Joseph O'Donnell's (2015) categories of what an anthropologist observes in a hospital ethnography, paying attention to what people do as well as to which artifacts are used (e.g., tools, paperwork, pictures, spatial layout), the symbolism attached to these, and the assumptions underlying people's beliefs and behaviors (the unconscious and taken for granted ways by which things are done).

Here, I follow the medical lives of thirty-six interns in two hospitals in the city of Puebla as they traverse their internship. I tell their stories of awareness, exhaustion, joy, and frustration. I also include the voices of their supervisors—the surgeons, obstetricians, and emergency room doctors who evaluate and teach them on their journey. These voices are most evident during formal *casos clínicos* (case presentations or grand rounds), an interactive event where trainees present a clinical case to their medical colleagues and discuss medical techniques, skills, differential diagnoses, and outcomes. These presentations sometimes take place in conjunction with an attending physician or resident. Residents, while still trainees themselves, are significant participants in the interns' transformation, and their voices are audible in this book. While interns are medical students, residents have completed their basic requirements for general practice and have passed a rigorous national examination before being accepted into a residency program.[3] They are above the interns on the medical hierarchy.

The social, economic, and racial distinctions between various groups in Mexico are very sharp and have been created by the historical processes that form the conditions for present-day mechanisms of exclusion. I explore how medical practice differs in private and public hospitals, which have vastly different facilities and patient loads, how the space constricts or encourages gendered ways of practice, and how men and women learn to navigate these sometimes hostile and violent spaces and interactions in different ways. Though much research has been done on medical socialization, I raise new questions. How is seemingly "invisible" knowledge about the practice of medicine transmitted to trainees? How does the (extra)ordinary form their medical self? How are physicians trained to think in certain ways about their patients? How do trainees cultivate their body to become expert? How does violence within and outside of the hospital impact the medical self?

PRACTICING MEDICINE WITHIN INTERSECTIONS OF RACE, COLOR, CLASS, AND GENDER

This book is about transformation—of medical students into medical selves. Though biomedicine is a global profession, it is taught, practiced, and experienced in local contexts (Good 1995b). I explain how interns embody a paradox. They are doctors in training, learning to wield new tools, language, and technology, sometimes with mixed results; they are exhausted from long work hours and little sleep; they are at the bottom of the medical hierarchy, doing the intensive, less recognized labor necessary for medical care. They do not feel like experts, yet from the moment they begin medical school they are referred to as "doctor," by both professors and patients alike. Their white coat, stethoscope, and newfound technical, linguistic, and sensory skills (Van Drie 2013) lend them an authority that they cultivate with each practice, transforming their sense of self. They help save patients' lives, deliver babies, and attend to victims of highway accidents. They sometimes do feel like experts. What I emphasize is the messy, complex, and nuanced nature of transformation, where interns not only have to acquire a monumental number of skills but do so against a backdrop of strict medical hierarchy within the hospital and a crumbling national medical system that inflicts violence upon them. This enskilment is fully immersive and "caught in the incessant flow of everyday life" (Pálsson 1994, 901)—it demands that interns be actively engaged with their environment, simultaneously learning and doing (Ingold 2000) rather than solely internalizing a stock of knowledge.

I explore the tensions and contradictions present in this transformation. I draw on frameworks of embodied learning (Downey 2010; Gieser 2008; Harris 2016; Prentice 2013) and of sensory enskilment in training (Pálsson 1994; Rose 1999; Van Dongen and Elema 2001; Van Drie 2013) to explain the fine-grained ways by which medical trainees learn new skills, practices, and bodily ways of attuning to/with the world around them (Csordas 1993, 138) as they inhabit their medical selves. Drawing on rich literature on reproduction, race, and gender (Andaya 2019; Davis 2019a; Gálvez 2019; Dixon 2015), I also address how medical transformation is conditioned by the broader political economy, such as Mexico's deep violence—structural, gender-based, obstetric, and caused by drug cartels. I attend especially to how the intersections and imbrication of class, gender, skin color, and ethnicity are acquired, enacted, reproduced, and perpetuated through medical bodies.

Mexico is a middle-income country with significant resource distribution issues in its health care: some medical centers are bereft of even basic supplies while others are extremely luxurious. Based upon ethnographic work in regional urban Mexico, I show how in the seemingly mundane practice of medicine, the most significant transformation takes place.

During most of the Mexican colonial period, doctors came from the Mexican upper classes and were required to be of "pure" (i.e., Spanish) ancestry. The patients and bodies on whom they practiced their skills, however, were primarily the impoverished and Indigenous (descended from the original inhabitants) populations who had little choice about how their bodies were treated by doctors.[4] Hospitals are colonial institutions that are sites for patient care and treatment while simultaneously being used for efforts at hygienic order, indoctrination, and civilizing projects (Anderson 2009; Zaman 2005). In these settings one finds significant historically based and prevalent class-based, gendered, and race-based distinctions. As Beatriz Reyes-Foster (2016; 2018) stated, aspects such as power, hierarchy, and inequality are very real within Mexican hospital wards, especially in public institutions, reflecting a persistent coloniality that maintains colonial relationships long after colonization ends.

To speak of race in Mexico is considered impolite. Instead, society takes great pains to deny, twist, and conceal the reality of racism and discrimination (Dulitzky 2005). Race in Mexico exists along a malleable social spectrum that incorporates color, class, power, and region (Braff 2013). Regardless of skin color, most of the population self-identifies as *mestizo* (mixture of white and Indigenous), though there are also Indigenous, Afro-Mexican, Asian, and white populations. The historical formal racialized structure of castes created during the colonial period was eventually abolished after independence. The country's leaders, aided by anthropologists (Ruiz 2001), promoted "assimilationist racism" (Gall 2004, 240) through a mestizo ideology. The assumption is that there is no racial discrimination because everyone belongs to the same "race" (Oboler and Dzidzienyo 2005).

However, the ambiguity of the concept of "mestizo"—which can range from more Indigenous to more European—hides profound discrimination (Ruiz

2001), which usually operates through a tight weave of social class and skin color (Aguilar 2013). People tend to, instead, euphemistically employ the term *cultura* when they talk about race (Ruiz 2001), assuming cultura to be a gentler word than race; however, as I will describe in future chapters, cultura is used in deeply discriminatory fashion against "problematic patients." This pigmentocracy (Telles, Flores, and Urrea-Giraldo 2015) socially stratifies based on color and is underlined by racial whiteness as an advantage (Nutini 1997), whereby whiteness is created through social processes of acquiring social or economic capital, and indexed by engaging in practices such as using reproductive technologies (Braff 2013; Roberts 2012). Like in Ugo Edu's (2019) work on racial aesthetics in Brazil, Mexico's race/class social ladder places at the top the populations who are perceived as whiter, more beautiful, and wealthier and at the bottom those perceived as darker, uglier, and more impoverished (see also Saldaña-Tejeda and Wade 2019).

This pigmentocracy is visible in current biomedical practice. Most present-day doctors continue to be drawn from middle-class and upper-class populations while the patients in public hospitals (where the bulk of medical training takes place) come from darker-skinned, poorer, and more disenfranchised populations. Mexico's socioeconomic racism becomes highly visible in contexts where things are "at stake"—such as in hospital wards where physician and patient interactions are fraught with the ever-present fear of risk of death. In hospital halls, you can hear some of the most unabashed criticism and racialized aesthetics against "those people," whoever they may be—teenage mothers, Indigenous people from the sierras, or "wily patients" (Bridges 2011, 227) who are seen to game the system by using more resources (medications, doctor hours, medical locations, etc.) than people believe they should or who do not follow the doctors' "medical common sense." For some doctors, knowing a patient's socioeconomic background is a shorthand to understanding where they had been treated previously—whether by a private doctor, a hospital, an auxiliary medical center, or a pharmacy—rather than to understanding their patients' lived experiences. Mexican hospitals become key places to unpack the enactment of institutional logic on the bodies of all actors involved.

TRANSFORMATIONS OF THE SELF

Like Seth Holmes, Angela Jenks, and Scott Stonington (2011, 106), I am fascinated by the question of "What kinds of people are formed through contemporary processes of clinical training?" This is a key question because a lengthy process like medical training that takes place in total institutions (Goffman 1961; Good 1994) like hospitals is not just about acquiring skills and knowledge, but is also about becoming something new: students become healers, experts, caregivers, decision-makers. Elizabeth Roberts (2016, 216) urged anthropologists to pay attention to the material realities of the practice of medicine, the broader political economy that shapes these practices, and how they both "produce certain kinds of deities in certain places and times." I am curious to understand how people behave when they are trained to have power over life and death. How is this process transformational to the interns' selves and identities?

Several anthropologists have focused on the way that biomedicine alienates patients' self from their body, making the person (and their illness) into an object (such as a patient or a case) able to be accessed by the medical gaze (Carpenter-Song 2011; Good 1994; Good and Good 1989; Young 1997). Mary-Jo and Byron Good (1989, 308) stated that these boundaries are also significant as medical students develop a professional self, wherein they must reorganize boundaries between themselves and patients, and struggle to resist being "swallowed up by medicine." As Tanya Luhrmann (2001, 533) suggested, the self is a cognitive schema and a bounded collection of conceptions and ideas that allow an individual to experience and think with the world. This sense of self is an introspective experience of "I" and exists in multiple ways: as one's relation to the physical environment, as one's interpersonal interactions, as something extended through time (our past selves and the selves we will become), as private (where we all have a sense of self that others cannot see), and as conceptual (consisting of the wealth of concepts, features, and traits that comprise oneself) (Luhrmann 2001).

I employ Rebecca Allahyari's (2000, 4) concept of moral selving, which she defined as the "work of creating oneself as a more virtuous, and often more spiritual, person," in order to understand the process of *medical* selving—which I define as the work of totally transforming oneself and not just a "situated identity." A medical self is created through both deliberate and passive forces wherein trainees must decide what *kind* of a medical self they hope to create through their practice of medicine (see Allahyari 1996 for a deeper analysis of moral selving). It is not solely about creating a new identity but is about re-creating one's entire sense of self—from the innermost recesses to the outermost skin—and is produced in the interactions with other people, objects, and spaces. My concept of medical selving is informed by Pierre Bourdieu's ([1977] 2000) habitus, by Tim Ingold's (2000) enskilment, and by scholars such as Tanya Luhrmann (2001), Thomas Csordas (1993), Nancy Scheper-Hughes and Margaret Lock (1987), and Elizabeth Carpenter-Song (2011) who connect questions of the self with embodiment and personhood. I suggest that medical selving is a deliberate process and runs deeper than simply identity. Bourdieu defined habitus as the ways certain collective dispositions, perceptions, thoughts, and actions become part of our body, which he conceptualizes as both the coordination of practices but also the practices of coordination. Habitus is the unconscious embodiment of ways of being into bodily practice and functions as a matrix of perceptions, appreciations, and actions (([1997] 2000, 83). Habitus is a product of history, producing collective and individual practices over time. It is physical rather than mental—that is, it is a cultivation of the body. Medical students deliberately cultivate a medical self through the use of tools (such as the stethoscope) or using medical terminology ("cephalea" rather than "headache") in their daily lives. They actively work to present themselves as professionals in their dress, manner, comportment, and attitude. They also passively acquire a medical self through the friction of their day-to-day interactions with the broader political economy structuring health care, the clinical hierarchies (rank and gender), the presentation of clinical cases, and the gradual acquisition of practical skills in diagnosis and treatment. This friction between active and passive medical selving shapes their transformation into expert medical selves.

Medical students learn in situated contexts; that is, through active participation and practice they become more experienced at what they do (Lave and Wenger 1991). In his work on enskilment and attunement in offshore sailors, Mike Brown (2017) suggested that "to become" is an ongoing practice and reoccurring process; it is a gradual sensory attunement to movement and perception. Trainees begin at the periphery of the action, gradually transforming and shifting into full participation as they gain mastery over their subject (Lave 2011). In the process they form a community of practice by engaging in the creation and acquisition of an identity and by distinguishing their practice and identity from others who are not part of the community. The body mediates this way of learning how to be in the world (Brown 2017). Medical interns learn new ways to see, speak, and write, and new hierarchies of valued knowledge, often as they struggle with new roles and identities (Good 2011). These formative acts (Good 1994, 81) are powerful ways of acting in these spaces that literally shape and reshape the body. Becoming a doctor is not just about reading about medicine or watching others doctoring; it is achieved through immersion and interaction that lead to a sense of "felt identity" (Brown 2017, 691). In the process, trainees come to "inhabit a new world" (Good 1994, 70) and transgress bodily boundaries.

I focus this research on high-stress medical wards, such as maternity and emergency wards, which are useful spaces to understand the transformation of medical students and their acquisition of a medical self because in these spaces people have to make quick decisions that can have life or death consequences for patients. Obstetrics wards, in particular, are spaces that reflect society's morals—about sexuality, about parenthood, and about bodily autonomy.

In cultivating a medical self in these spaces, interns do not simply learn new ways of knowing but also consciously learn new ways of being—how to attune their hands to become tools to measure the body's cavities or how to manage the hospital spaces and interactions. These ways of being are part of the process of embodiment; through practice, interns grow comfortable with their new environments and selves. At times these tools, such as the stethoscope, are emblematic of their status as doctors but also serve as tools to create their medical self—not a single intern I met ever forgot to wear their stethoscope on their body, whether around their neck or visibly tucked into a pocket of their white coat. Stethoscopes were not just a medical tool but an extension of their person, evident from their chosen decorations or color. As Tim Rice (2010) notes, the stethoscope is the "hallmark of a doctor" and allows medical students to enact certain dispositions as they develop a medical habitus through what Bourdieu calls structural exercises ([1977] 2000, 88). A stethoscope is emblematic of someone "medical." Even if the interns were not yet experts at auscultation (Harris 2016)—the science of listening to the body's noises—the stethoscope lent them an authority not possessed by others. Rice argued that on handling the stethoscope, medical students feel that they embody the professional habitus they aspire to have, as enacted by the doctors around them (see also Consejo and Viesca-Treviño 2008; Castro 2014).

One of the first steps in the development of the medical self is appearance—that is, wearing not only the stethoscope but also the white coat, white clothes, scrubs, and looking well put together. This part of the process begins from medical school where all students are required to wear a white uniform: men gel their hair and wear button-down shirts with ties and pants; women use makeup, jewelry, and professional clothes. In one conversation, a female medical student, who wore white scrubs under a white coat, with a white watch to match, noted that the correct white uniform was necessary "because it's part of [our] medical formation" and was a key way of visually demonstrating to others their discipline and conduct as physicians (Salhi 2016). As Ricardo stated in the quote included at the beginning of this chapter, when patients encounter doctors wearing the white coat "they entrust their lives to [the doctors]." When he and I met, he was in the first week of his internship and was still dazed about his new role. Yet he also acknowledged the almost-divine nature of skills of trained physicians (specifically surgeons), considering them to be so skilled that they are "like an extension of God's hand." Woven into his words is the idea that not anyone can have such skills; these skills take practice, they take time, and, however redundant it might sound, they take skill. Not everyone who goes to medical school will become godlike. Only the most skilled can have the audacity to extend God's divine powers into practice.

Interns spend one year in the hospital transforming into physicians through practice. These transformations occur over the course of the internship, through interactions with doctors who remind them of their duties, attitudes, and their identity as future doctors, as well as through micro-moments, such as Carlos painstakingly sawing through the full-body cast of a screaming toddler born with congenital hip deformities while he figured out how to wield the tool for the first time without it overheating. Or Rosa learning to do a colposcopy (a diagnostic procedure to examine the cervix for abnormalities, especially cancer) in the dysplasia department of the hospital: "On the first day, they let me see several colposcopies. The second day the resident explained to me [what he was doing].

And today they let me do it." Giggling, she added, "But I was still nervous." Rosa described how the procedure hurt the patient, and that she was scolded, not because of how she did the procedure but because she did it without direct supervision: "A [junior] resident was with me, but then he suddenly left and I was alone." She explained that the senior resident came in and saw her doing the procedure alone, with a patient who was complaining about the pain, and scolded her harshly. In these micro-moments, Carlos and Rosa learned not only how to wield technology and perform procedures, but also learned how to interact with patients and the importance of social position and hierarchy, their duties and responsibilities, and the role of punishment and obedience.

ETHNOGRAPHY IN MEDICAL SPACES

For this research I engaged in "studying up" (Nader 1972) through hospital ethnography; that is, I wanted to understand how the culture within medical institutions structures the lives of those who exist within them—whether as physicians, trainees, or patients. I employ a feminist ethnographic perspective (Davis and Craven 2016) by paying attention to power dynamics and questions of gender, race/color, and class, and listening to more silent and marginalized voices—even those practicing within spaces of privilege like hospitals. Hospitals have been primarily defined by researchers in two opposing ways: as bounded, island-like spaces (Coser 1962) that are separate from broader society and impose their own structure on bodies, or as "deceptively familiar" institutional spaces that can replicate and reproduce a society's key cultural norms and values, functioning with seemingly similar norms, bureaucracy, dress codes, or medical nomenclature across the world (Finkler 2004; Van der Geest and Finkler 2004, 1995). These are spaces where patients' needs, practitioners' skills, and technology's presence (or absence) are interwoven with broader bureaucratic and policy-based practices. Sometimes the state machine and the "hospital machine" are indistinguishable from each other, making it hard to understand where one ends and the other begins (Anderson 2009, 171). As Alice Street and Simon Coleman (2012) argue, hospitals are much more complex than these two extremes—they can be simultaneously bounded and permeable, where tight control is maintained over people's bodies and actions but also where new identities are constantly formed through interactions between people, technology, and space.

For patients, hospitals can be highly unfamiliar; patients feel they are between two states—well and unwell, mobile and immobile (Long, Hunter, and van der Geest 2008). Here one's former identity is left at the door with one's street clothing and belongings, and a new (albeit temporary) identity is created, clothed in hospital gowns, tethered to saline drips or catheters, and fed on a communal schedule. For practitioners, hospitals can also be both familiar and strange; practitioners also divest from their street identities, dressing in scrubs, white coats, and donning stethoscopes and IDs. In so doing, they take on new identities that are constantly being formed as they interact with each other, wield technology, and move through the hospital space. The space itself can be powerful in shaping the transformation of physicians. Navigating the tight space of a sterile field, entering into "staff only" spaces, or entering into the rooms of patients during medical rounds can serve as a powerful means of understanding their developing medical selves. Hospital ethnography is a method for understanding how all of these mutually articulated factors interact with each other, how individuals are shaped and constrained by them, how the global interplays with the local, and how they play out within a hospital setting. Because hospitals encompass nearly all facets of human life—from birth to death—events transpiring in their spaces have a much greater urgency than in everyday life, representing what Debbi Long, Cynthia Hunter, and Sjaak van der Geest have referred to as "a condensation and intensification of life in general" (2008, 73).

Within these spaces, medical practitioners provide varying forms of care, from highly involved to markedly detached. Different spaces have different "ethical locations" (Stonington 2012, 836); that is, different and unique value-laden and ethically based frameworks come into play in different spaces and govern what people can or cannot do (or should or should not do) there—where to give birth, where to die, or where to go for cancer treatment. Thus, when we apply methods of hospital ethnography, we have to take into account not only what people are doing or what values are guiding their actions, but also how these actions might vary in particular locations.

MEXICAN HEALTH CARE AND MEDICAL SYSTEM

Doctors have played an important role in Mexican politics and social life for more than two centuries, helping to develop and care for the health of the nation. In the first years after independence (early nineteenth century), the country's leaders yearned for the development of a national, Mexican form of medicine—not only in its practice but also in its innovation and teaching (Monteverde and Sánchez 2007). By the beginning of the twentieth century, despite being an independent nation for almost one hundred years, the social, economic, and political disparities created during the Mexican colonial period had become even more evident, which precipitated the 1910 revolution. The aim was to redistribute wealth and power into more people's hands, but the war ravaged the country, tearing apart much of the infrastructure and significantly damaging people's health.

The "social convulsions" (Jarillo Soto, Lemus, and Salinas Urbina 2011, 221) of the revolution resulted in an increase in the state's role in its population's welfare, which shifted the role of health and medical education from the periphery to the core of the country's emerging national identity. The government socialized care to the population and secured progress through modernization and industrialization

(Molyneux 2000). These ideas of social justice and equality became the substrate of the development of nationalized, bureaucratized, and institutional medicine—the intertwining of large public and private hospitals, social beneficence institutions, and medical schools. In this century we find the creation of some of the most significant Mexican institutions for social security, public welfare, health, and development: the *Secretaría de Salud* (Ministry of Health, established in 1917), the Mexican Institute for Social Security (known by its initials of IMSS, established in 1943, designed to provide health care to workers of private companies), and the Institute for the Security and Social Services for Workers of the State (ISSSTE, established in 1959, providing medical attention to civil servants and their families).[5] The creation of these state-sponsored health institutions concretized the ruling party's commitment to the health and well-being of the people (Soto Laveaga 2015), representing "the promise (if not the reality) of health care as a universal right" (Crowley-Matoka 2016, 20).

Medical formation continues to take place in tandem between medical schools and hospitals. Hospitals are crucial locations for the production of medical and scientific knowledge (Soto Laveaga 2015). In addition to their caregiving role, public hospitals have been significant sites for medical training, innovation, control, and practice. In their halls and wards, interns and residents formally learn the hands-on skills they need while also learning about patient care and hospital culture. Through practice, interns also learn in informal ways about the value of different populations: patients in public hospitals have less choice and their bodies are available for practice, but patients in private hospitals have more rights over their bodies and are not for practice.

The Mexican health-care system's coverage of its population has historically been fragmented. Just over 2 percent of the population is wealthy enough to afford private health insurance (Vargas-Bustamante and Méndez 2014). The remainder of the Mexican population are covered by public plans, although some who are able to afford it prefer to pay out of pocket for minor conditions rather than deal with the long waits and questionable care at public hospitals (Crowley-Matoka 2016; Wentzell 2013). About 50 percent of the population's health-care needs are either covered by IMSS or ISSSTE.[6] The rest of country's population is uninsured and falls outside formal labor sectors (e.g., rural, Indigenous, and geographically isolated populations, informal economy workers, and the urban poor); until 2004 the Secretaría de Salud provided them with basic health care (Frenk et al. 2006). In response to this hierarchical access to health care, in 2004 the country launched the Seguro Popular program, envisioned as a means to guarantee health-care access to marginalized populations and so to reduce the number of families affected by catastrophic health expenditures (Frenk 2006; Sosa-Rubí, Salinas-Rodríguez, and Galárraga 2011).[7] The program's detractors argued that medical care shifted from an integrated system that managed health through public funds to a neoliberal, free market–based system that emphasized patient responsibility for the benefit of the nation (López-Arellano and Blanco-Gil 2001; Homedes and Ugalde 2009; Reyes-Foster 2018). This program was cancelled in 2020 by the new president, Andrés Manuel López Obrador.[8]

Nationwide, the country has a ratio of 2.2 physicians for 1,000 people (World Health Organization 2019) and around four hospitals per 100,000 people, though the geographic distribution is highly unequal. This statistic places it within the Organisation for Economic Co-operation and Development (OECD) top ten nations with the lowest number of doctors (2020). Other countries in this category include India (0.8), South Africa (0.8), and the United States (2.6). Countries with a higher number of doctors includes Austria (5.2), Norway (4.8), and Germany (4.3) (OECD 2020). Almost 70 percent of all of Mexico's hospitals are private; the rest of the hospitals are public institutions intended to meet the medical needs of almost 98 percent of the population.[9] In 2014, the country spent approximately 6 percent of its gross domestic product on health, which by 2020 was estimated to be 2.5 percent; the state of Puebla spent just under 4 percent (Secretaría de Salud 2016).

For all these factors, Mexico is an excellent context in which to explore the question of medical transformation. The social and educational distinctions between physicians and most of their patients are stark. Hospital infrastructure is crumbling in many sectors, as health care budgets shrink yearly or are radically changed (Reyes-Foster 2018; Wentzell 2013; Crowley-Matoka 2016). Supplies can be quite limited in hospitals and clinics, where they run out of basic items such as gloves or suturing materials. Some public hospitals do not have any pain medication for women giving birth because their small supply is reserved for patients having cesarean deliveries. As Doctor Marco, one of the junior residents I met in the public hospital, said, they learn to "work with what [they] have rather than with what [they] would like to have."

Medical trainees, including both interns and residents, work long shifts during their training—some as long as thirty-six hours. Such long shifts have serious effects on trainees' acquisition of knowledge and their ability to practice skills. The impact they can have on patient health and welfare is also significant. By the end of their shift interns and residents are visibly exhausted, their clothes rumpled, their eyes red, their hair in disarray, their speech slower or slurred, and their motor skills affected. But most patients in public hospitals have no choice—they are treated by whoever receives their case. Throughout this book, I return to these political economic questions, and, like other ethnographers of hospital life (Crowley-Matoka 2016; Good 1995a; Hannig 2017; Livingston 2012; Prentice 2013; Reyes-Foster 2018; Wendland 2010; Wentzell 2013), I ask how these factors shape the ways that doctors practice. How can medical trainees transform into good doctors if they have no funds, no supplies, and no time to rest and reflect on practice?

As with any bureaucracy, medical care institutions in Mexico do not come problem free. Facing tremendous violence and inequities, Mexico continues to struggle to provide health care to its population. Many outstanding hospitals in the country rival the top medical institutions in high-income countries—but these are private institutions, where patients pay and physicians care. Public institutions, on the other hand, run the gamut from excellent research institutions with good patient care to substandard facilities with grueling hours for medical staff, high patient loads, and problematic delivery of medical care to patients. Within this substrate it is not surprising that problems have emerged, including lawsuits against physicians and large-scale protests by medical staff.

Only a tiny fraction of the Mexican population attends medical school. The relatively modest school fees make medicine a more accessible field of practice than in a country such as the United States.[10] Studies by the Mexican Institute for Competitiveness (Instituto Nacional Para la Competitividad [IMCO] 2018) show that the return on investment for students attending public and private medical schools is excellent and good, respectively. According to the National Statistics and Geography Institute (Instituto Nacional de Estadística y Geografía [INEGI]), the majority of medical students in Mexico come from middle and upwardly mobile classes; only 2.1 percent of the current medical population identify as speaking an Indigenous language (2014b). About 58 percent of physicians are women, and 42 percent are men, though most specialists are men. Almost 72 percent of physicians work in the public sector. On average, doctors earn a monthly income of 17,500 pesos (about $775 dollars), though this is a highly distributed system, with specialists and those working in the private sector earning several times this wage (IMCO 2018).[11] In 2016, the residents at Hospital Salud made approximately 8,100 pesos/month; many residents depended on their families for help. The interns at Salud made a small stipend of around 710 pesos/month, slightly more than what interns at Hospital Piedad made. A study by the medical school of the National Autonomous University of Mexico (Fernández-Ortega et al. 2016) found that the parents of their students were highly educated and worked in white collar jobs, with almost 50 percent of them having a bachelor's degree or higher.[12] My interlocutors tended to match this profile. Many had immediate family members who were engineers, physicians, or teachers; only a few had closer family members with blue-collar jobs, such as farming, plumbing, or working at small businesses. None identified as Indigenous, and most grew up in urban environments, primarily from Puebla but a handful from cities and towns in other states (Tlaxcala, Oaxaca, Guerrero, or Chiapas).

Medical school in Mexico is an undergraduate degree. Training extends over six years, with the first four spent in classrooms, where students learn the theory behind medical practice. The curriculum consists of a combination of basic (chemistry, physiology, pharmacology, etc.) and specialized (hematology, rheumatology, endocrinology, genetics, community health, surgery, bioethics, pediatrics, etc.) classroom training as well as preclinical practice in hospitals where students begin to learn skills such as taking samples, stitching basic sutures, and developing a bedside manner.

The interns on whom I focus in this book are students in their fifth year of medical school; they undertake a year-long rotation at a hospital, learning the skills, practices, and attitudes of medicine. Implemented in 1962, the internship had as its main aim the alignment of medical education with medical practice. Nationwide, internships are awarded based on a combination of grades and choice, and medical students usually have to decide between interning at a public or a private hospital, with each type having their own advantages and disadvantages. Within these broader categories exist other factors that influence students' choice—such as hospital size, location, patient base, or presence of residents. During the internship, interns learn the culture, life, and practices of a hospital. One resident described the internship as a phase "when one is a sponge," during which interns should acquire the basic ideas from each form of medicine and gain at least some useful skills. Interns rotate through the main areas of a hospital: pediatrics, gynecology, internal medicine, surgery, emergency medicine, and the intensive care unit (ICU). Each of these sections might have shorter subrotations within them; for instance, in pediatrics, interns might rotate through nursery, hospitalization, and newborn intensive care (NICU) where they gain more knowledge about different forms of medical practice and are reminded that clinical encounters need to consist of "inspection, interview, observation of the patient, examination, and exploration."

The sixth year is a mandatory year of social service, where *pasantes* are posted to underserved regions of the country to provide basic care to impoverished populations (Soto Laveaga 2013b; 2013c). At the completion of the social service, medical students are officially considered general practitioners. The year of social service was devised in the mid-1930s by presidential decree (later written into the constitution) and "tightly woven with post-revolutionary goals and rhetoric" (Soto Laveaga 2013c, 398). Most pasantes work in tiny, remote clinics as the sole physician, sometimes with the support of one or two nurses. Ideally the year of social service is meant to interweave medical education and medical practice for the health of the nation (Soto Laveaga 2013c), but the reality is that most urban-dwelling doctors are reluctant to serve rural populations, whom many consider to be socially or ethnically backward.

LIVING AND WORKING IN PUEBLA

The seeds for this research were planted in 2008 after I witnessed overt and seemingly intentional obstetric violence in a hospital in Puebla. The violence took the form of verbal and emotional abuse toward female patients as well as the presence of unnecessary obstetric interventions. The patients who were the objects of this violence were primarily low income, usually single mothers, or those who were reproducing outside of "the norm": considered too young, too old, or with too many children. The more I witnessed these interactions and the more I wrote about it (Smith-Oka 2013a, 2015), the more frustrated yet curious I became about its origins. Why did physicians act this way? Were they learning this behavior in medical school before they even set foot in a hospital? Were they learning these ways of interacting from their peers and work companions during their hospital years? Or, as Lydia Zacher Dixon (2015) suggested, was this violence somehow woven into the social fabric of Mexico—were the fissures of class, gender, and ethnicity so marked that it was inevitable that they would be enacted on patients?

I found myself looking back at some of my earlier research with rural Indigenous women in the state of Veracruz, who were racially and ethnically marked by economic and health institutions, to answer why some populations are classified as unfit mothers and citizens (Smith-Oka 2013b). Both these research strands—obstetric violence in hospital settings and structural violence in Indigenous communities—formed the substrate of my efforts to answer the puzzle of how these behaviors arise and are transformed, enacted, and experienced in the friction between institutions and the people who live within them and the patients they serve.

My research took place in the wards of two hospitals in the city of Puebla, located in the state of Puebla (figure 1). Almost everywhere you go in Puebla you see the phrase "*Que chula es Puebla,*" how sweet Puebla is. This phrase speaks to the city's juxtaposing identities—it is a sweet, delightful city, but with a violent history and highly segregated and stratified society. This disparity is reflected within the state of Puebla, which has a human development index of 0.7214, placing it twenty-ninth among the country's thirty-two states.[13] Much of the inequality is seen in people's purchasing power, education attainment, gender parity, and nutritional poverty (Programa de las Naciones Unidas para el Desarrollo [PNUD] 2014). Approximately 51 percent of the population lives on $197.26 a month (3,743.81 pesos) and 14 percent on $64.55 (1,225.16 pesos).[14] It is also rumored to be the city where top leaders of competing drug cartels have their families, which has created a détente of sorts. Until recently, it was considered a relatively safe city, though the past few years have seen an increase in kidnappings and murders.

Puebla is in a geographic halfway point between the port of Veracruz on the Gulf Coast and Mexico City in the center of the country, on a mostly flat valley, surrounded by some of the tallest and most striking volcanoes in the country, including the Popocatepetl, Iztaccihuatl, Matlalcueye, and Citlaltepetl. The Popocatepetl continues to be an active volcano, frequently ejecting dust and ash, much of which falls on Puebla itself (figure 2). This region is also prone to earthquakes, as evidenced by one on September 19, 2017, which caused the significant damage of several buildings in the city and surrounding villages. The nearby town of

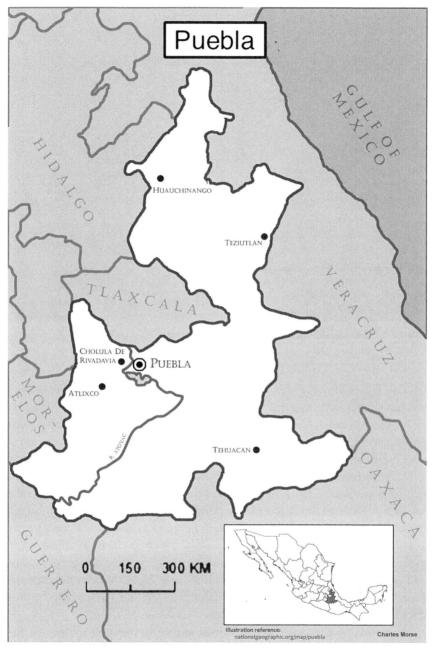

FIGURE 1. Map of the state and city of Puebla (illustrated by Charles Morse)

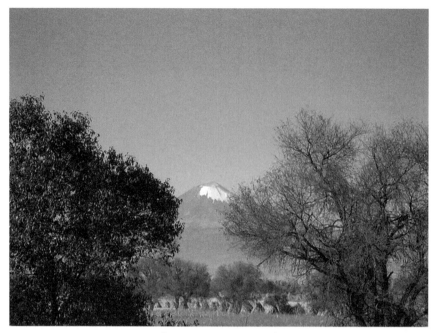

FIGURE 2. Popocatepetl volcano (photo by Pauline Smith)

Cholula is best known for its massive pyramid, atop of which sits a colonial-era church, visually depicting the violence of the colonial period.

Puebla was officially founded as a "social utopia" in 1531 where Indigenous populations and Spanish colonizers would supposedly live in harmony. However, the utopian plan failed. Colonizers were not eager to share the land or power with the original inhabitants, and the imagined harmony quickly vanished (Hirschberg 1979, 2). What remained and was subsequently developed over the following centuries was a planned, socially stratified city. It is now a bustling, dynamic industrial city of about 2.5 million people, 88 percent of whom identify as Catholic (INEGI 2010). Informal estimates suggest another 300–400,000 live in the larger metropolitan area, which includes large housing complexes, slums, and villages. Its city center, the *zócalo,* is listed as a United Nations Educational, Scientific and Cultural Organization (UNESCO) World Heritage Site and is also the city's religious and political center.

Poverty comingles with wealth in this large city (figure 3). Many of the colonial-era buildings have been converted into elegant hotels and restaurants, attracting thousands of tourists every year. Others hide dark tenement housing behind their colonial façade. Several of the streets are pedestrian only, drawing in both locals and tourists searching for bargains in the many shops. Food stalls selling *cemitas, churros, chalupas, esquites,* or *dulces poblanos* dot the sidewalks,

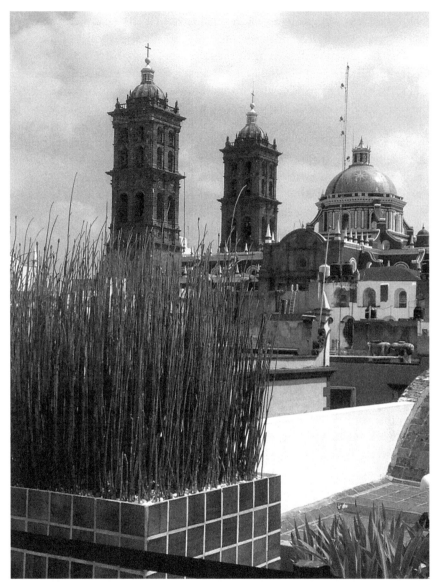

FIGURE 3. Rooftop view of Puebla's main cathedral

their delicious aromas interspersing with other urban scents. A man paints over the graffiti marring the black metal shutters of his store; the "hippies" hang out near the handicraft market, overtly selling woven bracelets and covertly dealing pot; tourists pose for selfies by the colorful "Puebla" sign next to the cathedral; a knife sharpener bicycles alongside the buses, *combis*, and Ubers on the road. The outskirts of the city are peppered with new high-rises, shopping malls, and bicycle overpasses, while the roads to get to them have snarled traffic, street vendors, tourists, and beggars. Beyond these outskirts lie small villages and hamlets, many of which have been swallowed up by the urban sprawl.

The social and economic stratification is visible in the health facilities (figures 4 and 5). There are many excellent hospitals in the city, both public and private, but there are also many that have high iatrogenic rates (doctor-caused problems), causing more harm than good to their (usually impoverished) patients. Some of the large private hospitals are humorously referred to as "hotels" because of the extreme luxury of their lobbies and patient rooms. There are also many public hospitals that are markedly understaffed and with decrepit facilities—stained medical gowns, third-hand equipment, and poor plumbing. One of the newest public hospitals in the state is a trauma and orthopedics hospital located near the interstate highway.

Just under half of the city's population has no formal health insurance (INEGI 2014a) and less than 5 percent of the population receive privately based medical care. At the national level, the state of Puebla ranks at twenty-two (out of thirty-two) in the number of general practitioners and twenty-seventh in the number of specialists (Secretaría de Salud 2016). Despite some of these dire statistics, which indicate the structure of health care distribution and provision across the country, my interlocutors tended to think of their ways of doing medicine as effective. As one person put it, "We're actually not that badly off clinically" in Mexico.

A key part of my research in 2016 was my research assistant Megan. She was my former student, had lived in Puebla, and was planning on becoming a physician. She participated significantly in data collection and was a wonderful sounding board during my time in the field. As part of hospital ethnography, I drew from both qualitative and quantitative approaches in my methods, combining classic qualitative ethnographic inquiry and quantitative survey methods with a total of ninety-five participants (interns, residents, and physicians) and many hours of "deep hanging out" (Geertz 1998) and observations of their lives in hospital. My primary intern interlocutors were in their early twenties, most residents were in their late twenties, and many—though not all—of the physicians were between thirty and fifty years of age. I established a close rapport with the interns. We ate meals together in the staff cafeteria, I hung out with them in their hospital residence, and I followed them into simple and complex procedures in the emergency, obstetrics, and surgical wards.

In these hospital spaces the interns' interactions with their peers and with the physicians and nurses noticeably shaped their practice. I heard the praise they received for good work, and the reprimands to which they were subject when they did not know the case or the technique. I witnessed them practicing for case presentations to their peers and supervisors and the grilling they received from senior doctors when their lack of knowledge was apparent. By witnessing their

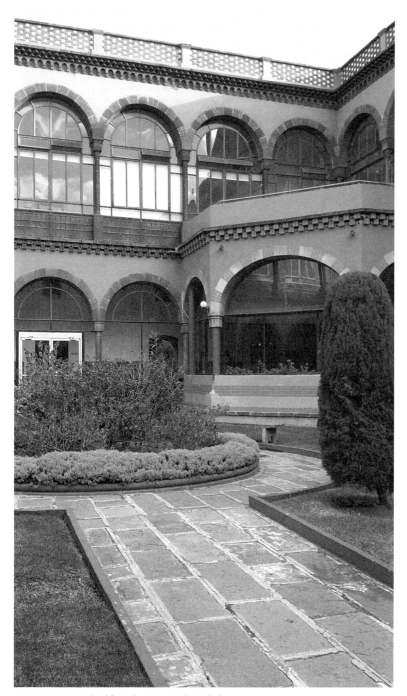

FIGURE 4. Main building for Hospital Piedad

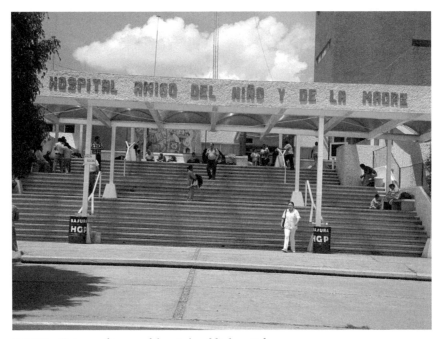

FIGURE 5. Entrance for one of the city's public hospitals

lives, I began to understand that to be a medical student was more than just knowing "stuff" about medicine. It was a gradual and detailed transformation of the medical self and learning to inhabit a new form of bodily practice. To transform within a space that exists in a resource-poor setting is not linear nor straightforward; it took creativity, fortitude, and endurance to cope with the rigors of medicine as a practice (figure 6).

I lived and worked in Puebla during various field seasons between 2008 and 2016, though the bulk of the data for this book came from a five-month period in 2016. In this book I refer to the two hospitals where I did my research as Hospital Piedad and Hospital Salud. Hospital Piedad is a small, private hospital run by a religious organization. Housed in part in a beautiful red brick building built in 1885, it is located in the historic city center. The three-storied older building contains the outpatient care, administrative offices, chapel, cafeteria, and trainee residences; it surrounds an open-air central courtyard with a few bushes and an old well that the interns claimed houses the ghost of an old friar. A tall minaret hints at the Islamic influence on Spanish colonial architectural styles. An adjoining, newer four-storied building contains the inpatient hospital services (surgery, pediatrics, intensive care unit, obstetrics, and emergency departments). The hospital's patient base is primarily middle-income, as evidenced by the number of insurance posters in the passages and waiting rooms that advertise competitive rates for procedures such as cesareans. In 2016 it had forty beds, approximately

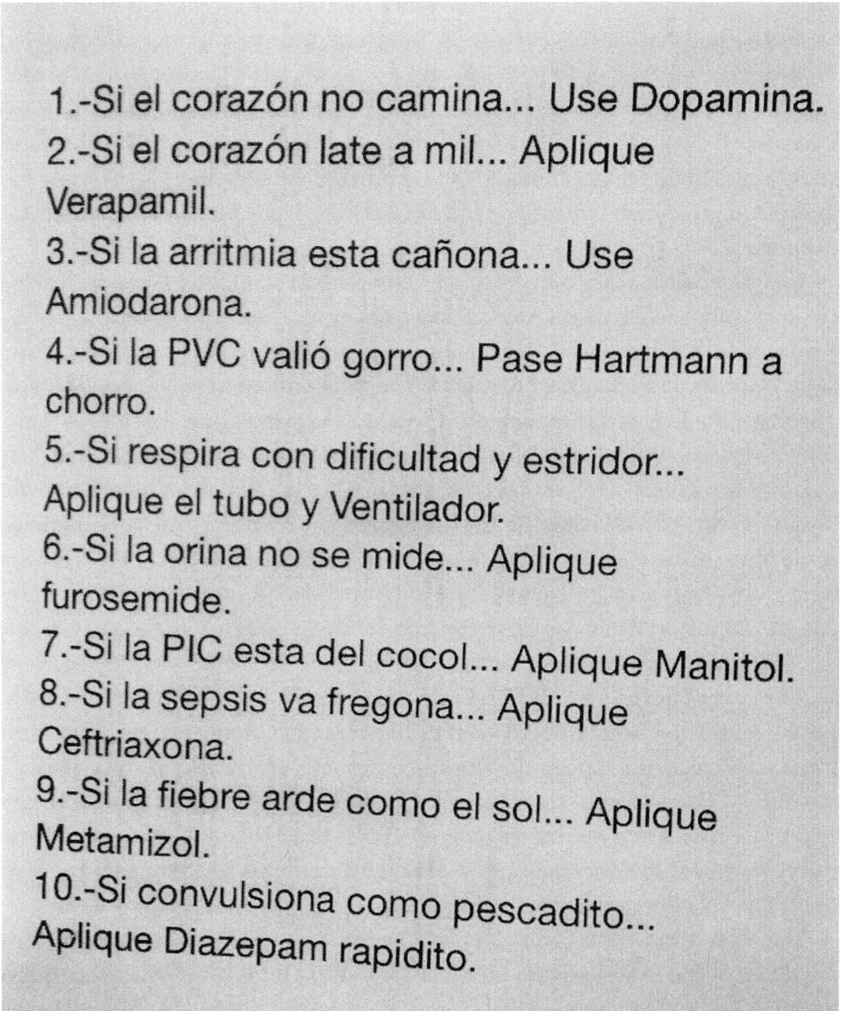

1.-Si el corazón no camina... Use Dopamina.

2.-Si el corazón late a mil... Aplique Verapamil.

3.-Si la arritmia esta cañona... Use Amiodarona.

4.-Si la PVC valió gorro... Pase Hartmann a chorro.

5.-Si respira con dificultad y estridor... Aplique el tubo y Ventilador.

6.-Si la orina no se mide... Aplique furosemide.

7.-Si la PIC esta del cocol... Aplique Manitol.

8.-Si la sepsis va fregona... Aplique Ceftriaxona.

9.-Si la fiebre arde como el sol... Aplique Metamizol.

10.-Si convulsiona como pescadito... Aplique Diazepam rapidito.

FIGURE 6. A list of tongue-in-cheek, rhyming mnemonics created by the interns: 1. If the heart doesn't spring, use Dopamine; 2. If the heart is beating at a thousand mil, apply Verapamil; 3. If the arrhythmia is freakin' [awful], use Amiodarone; 4. If the CVP (central venous pressure) has gone to hell, Hartmann's must gush well; 5. If the breathing is difficult and strident, put in a tube and ventilate; 6. If urination is meager, use furosemide; 7. If the ICP (intracranial pressure) is awful, use Manitol; 8. If the sepsis is freakin' [gruesome], apply Ceftriaxone; 9. If the fever burns like the sun, apply Metamizol; 10. If they convulse like a fishy, apply Diazepam real quickly.

seventy-five physicians on staff, and twenty-two interns. At the end of my field-work, the hospital underwent a week-long recertification. Posters on the wall excitedly reminded staff to be ready and prepared: "2016 Certification. Prepare and Act. Let's go for the 2016 Certification!"[15] Interns were cautioned to be on their best behavior and keep a low profile, and they were handed manuals to study and told that if questioned by the external reviewers they had to know the answers for practices such as proper hand washing or the protocols for filling out paperwork.

Hospital Salud is a public hospital belonging to the ISSSTE system whose civil-servant patient base is lower-middle and low income. In 2016, it had 130 beds. It is surrounded by several low-income communities and is located close to a large Walmart and other big box stores. The main entrance is quite nondescript. The first time I visited I wondered if I was at the wrong place. It is located on a tiny road, squashed between other buildings along with small businesses such as taco and torta stalls, copy shops, and a *funeraria* (a funeral parlor) that serve the hospital's workers and patients. The hospital is spread over a series of buildings, some more institutional-looking than others. During my research, the hallways were always busy with patients waiting to be attended. A mural is painted on the entrance's inner wall that depicts the medical systems of China, India, and Greece, the Hippocratic Oath (in Spanish), pre-Hispanic medicine, and the current social issues of poverty and health in Puebla, culminating with the state hospital system and its governing board. Murals like this exist in most large public hospitals in Mexico, portraying the hopes and aspirations of the nation's goals of modernity, interweaving science, medicine, and social revolutions (Soto Laveaga 2015). Gabriela Soto Laveaga has suggested that these "massive canvasses" allow the government to concretely show what they are doing for their country's (or state's) population's welfare (2015, 276).

The obstetrics ward is in an older building that also houses pediatrics, includ-ing the neonatal intensive care unit (NICU). It has thirty-five beds to attend to between five and ten births a day; about 60 to 70 percent of these are cesarean deliveries.[16] It has white walls and grayish floors, and is lit with bare, bright fluo-rescent ceiling lights. Along the passage walls hang large posters of women breast-feeding their babies; one poster depicts several babies of all skin colors sitting side by side with the wording "Exclusive breastfeeding prevents pregnancy dur-ing the first six months after birth and favors physical and emotional develop-ment." A sign on one of the doors reads "Area free of baby bottles," indicating that this is a "Baby Friendly Hospital." Additional banners and posters on the walls list the rights of patients, physicians, nurses, and administrative personnel. Other posters list the hospital's mission, vision, and code of ethics and values.

Hard plastic chairs, their white paint chipped in many places, are the sole places for patients to sit while they wait. The hallways resonate with the noise from people's chatter, coughs, or laughter. Wails from babies and children punctuate the hum of noise. The air smells faintly of antiseptic. The passages in the medical personnel–only areas, especially those leading to the labor and delivery wards, were darker and more decrepit, with several of the wings closed off and no longer in use. Public records suggest that in 2016 the hospital had almost 400 physicians and residents (across all specialties) and fifty interns (Datos Abiertos 2016). I obtained basic demographic data on most of the interns, but only observed the lives and practices of eight of them in-depth, as I will describe.

During my first foray into the obstetrics sterile area of Hospital Salud, I got lost. Doctor Rafael, the third-year resident who had invited me into the area to observe a hysterectomy, pointed to the women's changing room, saying, "I'll see you soon," and disappeared into the men's room. I changed hurriedly into the clothes required within sterile spaces (scrubs and disposable boots, surgical cap, and face mask), assuming I would see him back out in the passage so he could show me the way into the surgical area. I waited in the passage for several minutes, holding the plastic bag with my street clothes, walking up and down the completely empty passage and peering around corners to other empty passages to see if I had somehow missed the door that I could go through. But I saw nothing. Desperate and wondering what my next move would be, I saw Iker walking down toward the men's changing room. An intern who over time would become a close interlocutor, Iker asked me what I was doing there. When I explained, he looked at me curiously and told me the changing room had access into the sterile transfer. Feeling rather stupid, I walked back into the changing room and immediately saw the very obvious door leading to the transfer. Leaving my street clothes on one of the changing room benches, I walked through and sat on the tiled bench separating the sterile from the nonsterile areas, putting my paper boots over my shoes. I had not entered a sterile hospital area for two years. Not wanting to appear even more stupid, I tried to get the boots on as quickly and professionally as possible. I was not successful. Iker came out of the men's changing room and saw that I was not yet fully clothed in the sterile materials. He helped me with one of the boots, tying it expertly, explaining the importance of covering the legs of my scrubs trousers so I would not drag anything into the area or collect anything nasty onto my own clothes. In the time it took me to figure out the second boot, adjust my hair under the surgical cap, and place the facemask on, Iker had already dressed and disappeared down the passage of the sterile area.

My primary focus and interest for many years has been in the anthropology of reproduction, and I gravitated toward the obstetrics and gynecology practices in each hospital. At Hospital Salud I observed and interviewed the eight interns doing their rotation in obstetrics and gynecology. I followed them into various procedures—such as vaginal births, cesarean deliveries, or hysterectomies. I interviewed them as they carried out their duties as interns—examining patients, entering information into the patient records, and running samples to the laboratory. I saw how Rosa was taught to open surgical packets, or how fearful Evelyn became during a cesarean delivery when she was the scrub technician (handing surgical tools to the surgeons). I saw how Kevin's easygoing nature and evident skills made him a natural leader among his peers.

Because Hospital Piedad had only twenty-two interns, I interviewed all but one of them (the exception was an intern whose external rotations at other hospitals never allowed our time to coincide). I spent a significant amount of my time in the emergency ward where I followed interns such as Gabriel, Carlos, and Victoria into the curtained cubicles as they attended to the needs of their patients. I also observed the surgery ward for obstetrics and gynecology, where I looked on as Aarón and Sebastián were instructed as surgical assistants in cesarean deliveries. I hung out in the residence, as Julieta filled out patient history forms while she watched video recipes online, Lucero prepared a PowerPoint for a case presentation, and Emilio and Mauricio dozed on a bunk, their legs dangling over the side. I was in the hospital overnight when the bus accident occurred and witnessed the strain and exhaustion of the interns—but also how humor and lighthearted interactions helped them to handle the strain.

Ethnography in Mexico is always a deeply personal and humbling experience for me. As a visitor in these medical spaces I was expected to dress in scrubs and white coat, despite not being a physician. This medical drag allowed me entry into spaces I would never have seen as a layperson, but it also created an unbridgeable divide between the patients and me, as they assumed I was one of the clinicians who held their lives in my hands. Every time I donned these medical uniforms, I felt I was in costume, and I uncomfortably wore the clothes as a form of performance of medicine without having any of the skills or abilities of actual clinicians. As an Anglo-Mexican, I straddle three worlds—the Mexico where I grew up, the South American/Anglo of my parents' background, and my years of living and working in the United States. I am in many ways a clear outsider—phenotypically and professionally (I am an anthropologist, not a physician)—which sometimes fosters connection with people who warm to my inquiries about their lives, and sometimes alienates people who assume I am an entitled, foreign interloper. And yet I am also an insider—I am culturally Mexican and linguistically able to blend into the local terms and slang.

Embodying these occasionally juxtaposing identities provided me entry into certain domains of interaction and allowed me to see multiple facets of the lives I was researching. My non-medical background meant that in terms of skills I was lower than any trainee—I knew virtually nothing that was valued (except perhaps speaking English). I paid close attention to how people moved in these spaces and how they interacted with each other in order to learn the hierarchy, to place one's self within sterile spaces, to enter and exit locations, and many other skills. I had several faux pas over my time doing research—including being scolded once or twice for forgetting important rules of behavior. Over time I grew more practiced, though never expert.

THE BOOK AND ITS CHAPTERS

The five ethnographic chapters that follow this introduction provide facets of the story of how knowledge and concepts about medicine are embodied and how these forces shape the transformation of trainees into experts. In Chapter 1, "Women Can't Be Trauma Doctors," I analyze the ways that race, color, gender, and class have affected the history of medicine in Mexico and shape current medical practice, particularly how hospital spaces can be hostile to women, how men are trained with a harder hand, and how women are often compelled to employ a "dirty trade" with male attending physicians and residents that capitalizes on their beauty to gain entry into these spaces. Chapter 2 addresses the internal and external forms of violence affecting medical training and practice. I describe how doctors in Mexico have used protest as a means to push back against society's expectations of them while simultaneously being deaf to the presence of violence within medical spaces—such as teaching by humiliation or the excessive use of punishments. Chapter 3, "The Soul of the Hospital," introduces the reader to the life of a medical intern in the hospital ward, paying attention to how the artifacts used, the values espoused and practiced, and the invisible assumptions in these spaces and interactions develop the medical self in the ordinary spaces and experiences as well as in the extraordinary.

Chapter 4 examines obstetric violence—which is the abuse and mistreatment of women during labor—and shows how female clinicians can internalize some of the violent structures of medicine and reproduce them in these settings; they can be both victims and perpetrators of gender-based violence. Chapter 5, "The Body Learns," brings the reader deeper into obstetric medicine and analyzes three cases—a cesarean delivery, a vaginal birth, and a stillbirth—to answer how medical senses are embodied in these spaces, and how reproduction brings into sharp focus society's disappointments and desires. Here I address the ways that interns embody some of the values of medicine in their techniques and practices.

Following these ethnographic chapters, in the book's conclusion I explain the interns' emerging identity as almost-gods. I contextualize the multiple forces affecting their medical selves as they take their first steps into the profession of medicine in an increasingly changing medical structure. Although my research began as an inquiry into why doctors were sometimes abusive to their patients and why they sometimes perpetuated broader racist or gendered structures in their patient care, the more time I spent in the medical spaces with medical providers, the more I began to understand the problematic structures within which they attempted to provide medical care. I grew to respect them in ways I never anticipated.

1 · WOMEN CAN'T BE TRAUMA DOCTORS, AND OTHER GENDERED STORIES OF MEDICINE

Sometimes orthopedic [surgeons] request male [assistants] for the surgeries. Why? Because these surgeries are difficult and hard [*pesadas*]. They involve heavy lifting and strong hammering, bang, bang, bang. So maybe women are more delicate. Though there are female orthopedic surgeons …, I feel that it's harder for women to be physicians.

—Gabriel, intern at Hospital Piedad

We're writing up notes, and they sit really close, … and they start to invite you to go on a date, or to go to the movies.… So, it's like an uncomfortable feeling.

—Rosa, intern at Hospital Salud

As a man you are better able to *aguantar* [endure]. Because a girl stresses out.

—Aarón, intern at Hospital Piedad

In this chapter I deepen the analysis of the development of a medical self by focusing on the complex ways that gender inheres in the body. I delve into a brief history of medicine in Mexico to illustrate how deep-seated many of these medical structures are and how extraordinary the presence of women is in these medical spaces. A frequent aphorism among my interlocutors was "women can't be trauma doctors." The rationale for this belief was based on a perceived binary: female weakness and male strength. The prevailing adage among my interlocutors was that female doctors were as technically and intellectually competent as men, but they said that women were more likely to be emotional, sensitive, or physically weak. This perceived weakness allegedly made women more *delicadas*—delicate—so they were treated differently from men in how they were scolded, in what they traded to be invited into procedures, in what gendered assumptions were made about their abilities, and in the ways their bodies belonged (or not) in medical spaces.[1] Being delicadas also made women targets of sexual and gender-based harassment, which they learned to manage in order to survive their training. Men's perceived strength, conversely, often meant a greater need to perform masculinity in the face of harsh scolding. What was especially noteworthy was how prevalent these gendered ideas were throughout the hospitals, among both men and women.[2]

Victoria had been prompted to enter medicine for vocational and pragmatic reasons—when she was a teenager her grandmother fell sick, and Victoria would accompany her to the hospital. She discovered there her fascination for the profession while also realizing that "one needs a physician in the family." She was one of my most active interlocutors at Hospital Piedad, frequently seeking out opportunities for me to witness interns' medical training, and she was always accommodating to the many questions I had about their medical lives. She was an assertive, hardworking, and very well-liked intern, who was not afraid to speak her mind, whether to her peers or senior doctors during medical rounds or to me during conversations and interviews about training. Her round face was framed by dark hair, glossy and smooth, which she often tied back into a ponytail, as required for all female staff. Like other female interns, she took great care of her appearance, making certain her eyebrows were trimmed and that she wore makeup. Her medical ensemble also included small silver earrings and a silver pendant of a Catholic saint.

During the many months of our acquaintance, Victoria always struck me as a feminist, which is why it came as a surprise when in one of our interviews she said that women were less capable than men of being trauma and orthopedics doctors.

> I think it is mostly perhaps because of strength. . . . I've seen that trauma surgeons . . . are tall, super tall, like that. And when a woman wants to be a trauma surgeon, you say, "Yikes! How is she going to pull a leg and, I don't know, put in screws, and such?"
>
> [I asked her whether she thought women were not strong.]
>
> Sure [they are]. I have seen female trauma surgeons who are thin, thin, and tiny, tiny. And, I don't know, maybe it is harder for them, but they do manage, right? But I do think that [those factors] do influence. Because women are probably more delicadas, they prefer specialties like dermatology or hematology.

It was evident that there was a particularly marked gendered nature to practice, with some specialties considered to be "male" and others "female." As Nicolás, an intern at Hospital Salud, said, "Dermatology is kind of more related to beauty, and women are kind of more attuned to that, right? Like, they take care of themselves, use creams and that kind of stuff."

Most of my female interlocutors emphasized how frequently they had been told by surgeons that "We need a male intern" as a reason for not being allowed entry into a surgery. They stated that some specialties such as orthopedics are "dominated by men" and are noticeably *machista* (sexist). This dominance was numeric (with more men than women accepted into certain specialties), structural (with some surgical residencies not accepting women), organizational (with male surgeons preferentially teaching male interns), or even patient based (with patients tending to seek out male surgeons for care). The interns' beliefs were illustrative of a larger pattern about how perceptions of gender, practice, abilities, and personalities were intertwined within medical training.

Using these gendered perceptions as a starting point, in this chapter I explore the ways by which gender inheres in the body of medical trainees.[3] To do so I draw from Nessette Falu's (2019) work on Brazilian gynecology to inquire how medicine reproduces gendered social norms and from Joan Cassell's (2000) research on the embodiment and intertwining of gender and the medical body among female surgeons in the United States. Falu's work addresses the racial prejudice in Brazilian gynecology that reproduces multiple "interlocking oppressions," including racism, genderism, sexism, homophobia, colorism, and classism (2019, 696). Cassell investigated surgical embodiment in general, and the embodiment of female surgeons specifically. She asked whether the body of a female doctor responds to the body of patients in the same way as a male body would, whether her body carries the same meaning to colleagues, nurses, and trainees, and whether the female medical body is perceived to be different.

I use my participants' stories of gendered medicine as an entry point into a discussion of the embodied and spatial forms of practice in hospital wards. Women physicians were described as more naturally tied to their biology than men and were not considered to have the fortitude for strong medicine. Men, on the other hand, because of their perceived ability to rise above their biology (Ortner 1974) were seen to be free to develop and master these cultures of medicine. They were perceived as stronger and able to tolerate harsher training, referred to as *mano dura*—heavy/hard hand.

AGAINST NATURE: WOMEN OUT OF SPACE

The education of women was a topic of heated debate and polemic in the late nineteenth and early twentieth centuries, particularly whether women should be educated, what would happen to society if they surpassed men, and whether they should simply stay home and carry out activities that were more in line with their "nature." High-status professions were the realm of men, which reflected the preferred characteristics of middle-class men who labored in them, such as being rational, unemotional, physically robust, scientific, willing to sacrifice, mentally tough, aggressive, and committed to long hours (Adams 2010; Demaiter and

Adams 2009). The idea of masculinity became contingently associated with emotional distance (McElhinny 1994). Women in these professions served as support—as assistants or nurses—and were actively excluded from higher status work because they were considered to be frail, emotional, dependent, and less committed to employment (Adams 2010). Barriers to women entering these professions were not only about "doors and minds being closed" (Davies 1996, 669) but also reflected the embedded values of a masculinist worldview.

It was only in the mid-nineteenth century that women finally gained entrance into medical schools. Even so, once admitted, they often faced hostility and opposition from their male counterparts. Women such as Elizabeth Blackwell or Mary Edwards Walker in the United States (earning their degrees in 1849 and 1855, respectively) opened the door for other women to attend university, such as Rebecca Lee Crumpler, who became the first African American female physician. Anandibai Joshi from India, Kei Okami from Japan, Sabat Islambooly, a Kurdish Jewish woman from Syria (Kosambi 1996; Werman and Woolf 2013), and Rebecca Cole, an African American woman (Epps, Johnson, and Vaughan 1993), all received their training at the Women's Medical College of Pennsylvania in the United States. In increasing numbers, women in Latin America directly confronted the state, beginning the process of dismantling patriarchal authority in legal, professional, and personal spheres—a process that continues to this day (Dore 2000). The first female doctor in Mexico was Matilde Montoya, who received her degree in 1887; she had previously trained as a midwife—the only medical profession, besides nursing, open to women—and was allowed into medicine by presidential permission.[4] She was followed by other women, including Herminia Franco Espinosa who in 1915 became the first woman to graduate from the medical school in Puebla.

Women who pursued a medical education in Mexico were called "shameless and dangerous" (Arias Amaral and Ramos Ponce 2011, 467) or "depraved to want to see the cadavers of naked men" (Carrillo Esper et al. 2015, 163) (my translations). Public opinion was divided into those who called them immoral and those who thought they were heroic (Jaramillo-Tallabs 2010). Many people were aghast at what they perceived as social disintegration (see Molyneux 2000). Others believed that women's nature and "delicate constitution" made them unable to labor in clinical settings, especially surgery where they would be confronted by real anatomy. Such arguments stated that if women did engage in higher education their weak constitution would not allow them to proceed, and they could collapse from nervous exhaustion (Briggs 2000). Still others falsely predicted that in two generations women would no longer be mothers or wives because becoming professionals would eradicate their femininity, essentially masculinizing them.[5]

Medical training necessitates rapid acculturation, homogenization, and conformity into the profession, including its culture and behaviors, in the process neutralizing one's former self (Babaria et al. 2012). This process creates the substrate for the medical self to develop more fully and concretely. Though the medical profession worldwide is rapidly feminizing, medical students continue to be socialized to be gender neutral (i.e., male as an unmarked category), and it is assumed that medicine is value-, culture-, and gender-free (Riska and Novels-kaite 2008). The reality, of course, is that health-care professions are un-neutral, with gender, race, color, and class beliefs interwoven into the professional work, identity, and perceptions of practice (Adams 2010; Wendland 2010), which I will discuss in future chapters.

In Mexico, although women make up over 50 percent of medical students (Cortés-Flores et al. 2005), the proportion radically changes for further education and specialization; on average 1.7 more men than women work as specialists (62.6 percent of specialists are men) (Heinze-Martín et al. 2018). Surgical specialties have a much lower proportion of women, with some like urology or orthopedics having only 2.9 percent and 3.4 percent of female surgeons, respectively (Cortés-Flores et al. 2005). These old boys' clubs reproduce institutionalized patterns of a male worldview "in ways not always visible or obvious" (Biswas 2019). Women may also be subordinated through the deployment of gendered language; for instance, female interns and trainees are more likely than their male peers to be called *hija* (child) by male physicians, or a female doctor's title is omitted by others, subordinating female authority and expertise (Files et al. 2017).

In order to understand some of the stratified and spatial dynamics present in contemporary hospitals and appreciate how these larger contexts have shaped the identity, learning, and practice of Mexican physicians (Soto Laveaga and Agostoni 2011), a brief historical and social context to the medical system in Mexico is necessary.

COLONIAL HOSPITALS

When the Spaniards colonized the area subsequently known as New Spain in the early 1500s, some of the first buildings they founded were hospitals. These hospitals were owned and managed by the Catholic church and were a central part of the brutal colonizing effort during the first few decades after contact (Martínez Barbosa 2007).[6] In later centuries Puebla was known as the "Mexican Rome," not only because of its many stone buildings but also because more than half of them were owned by the church (Robles Galindo 2012).

The first medical school was established in 1579 in Mexico City. It reflected colonial ideologies (Ramírez-Ortega 2010): its (male) students were required to have "pure" European blood[7] (Rodríguez 2007; 2010), and its curriculum was formally based on humoral Galenic and Hippocratic medicine, though it also began to appropriate Indigenous concepts into its practice (Sanfilippo 2007). For almost two centuries, this was the only university to offer medicine as a field of study in New Spain.

In 1770, the Royal College of Surgery was inaugurated to improve surgical training in the colony by introducing new European anatomical approaches, surgical techniques, and models of understanding the body and disease (Ramírez-Ortega 2010). The Surgical College was housed in the Hospital Real de Naturales—the Royal Hospital for Natives. This partnership between university and hospital rapidly increased understanding of human anatomy, but it did so while reflecting the colonial worldview of racial hierarchy and worth. Such hierarchies embed within them notions of idealized, hegemonic masculinity associated with racism and colonial power (Kanitkar 1994).

Within the racialized hierarchy of the colonial order, Indigenous populations were categorized as inferior humans—below those of Spanish or *mestizo* (mixed) ancestry—and when they died in this hospital, they were usually autopsied (Romero-Huesca and Ramírez-Bollas 2003). In this way, medical knowledge in New Spain was literally carved from the bodies of those without power. In many ways, this practice continues to be true in Mexico, as public hospitals that serve impoverished populations are the primary training grounds for hands-on practice.[8]

By the end of the eighteenth century, medical training began shifting power beyond the confines of the country's capital city (Ramírez-Ortega 2010) and opening up learning opportunities to students who were not of "pure" Spanish blood. With this change, so too practices changed of whose bodies were allowed entry into medical learning spaces and in what capacity—not just as cadavers, but also as practitioners.

The nineteenth century was one of the most turbulent centuries of Mexico's modern history: independence from Spain in 1821; the Mexican–American War from 1846 to 1848; the French Intervention and the subsequent reign of Emperor Maximilian from 1861 to 1867; and the rise of liberalism, republicanism, nationalism, and modernization personified by presidents such as Benito Juárez and Porfirio Díaz (see also Reyes-Foster 2018).[9] People's health suffered from the ravages of conflict and displacement, from deep structural poverty, and from epidemics. The Mexican state's intervention in health matters increased (Agostoni 2003), regulating medical education, research, and practice. Influenced by European approaches to medicine, including antiseptic and sterile measures as well as anatomy and the dissection of cadavers (Fajardo-Ortiz 2002; Rodríguez-Sala 2005), Mexican medicine also drew from new paradigms of scientific and positivist perspectives and approaches. Mexico transformed into a "modern" and "hygienic" nation through inculcating responsibility in its populations as well as emphasizing order and hygiene in public spaces and private lives (Agostoni 2007).

The existing hospitals were seen as outdated colonial holdovers (Robles Galindo 2012), and they were replaced by more "modern" secular medical institutions (Fajardo-Ortiz 1999). No longer considered an art, medicine became increasingly professionalized (Robles Galindo 2012), and its practitioners gained greater prestige in society, forming part of the intellectual elite.[10] As historian Gabriela Soto Laveaga (2013b) states, physicians held both actual positions of power and moral and symbolic power in bringing science and modernity to all corners of Mexico through their health-care role. As in other parts of the world, medicine in Mexico became spatially connected to the hospital and clinical wards. A discursive shift went hand in hand with the clinical gaze: doctors shifted from seeing the patient as a whole to seeing them as a series of component parts that were subsequently compared and analyzed to reach a diagnosis (Foucault 1973). Clinical medicine was not only medicine taught "alongside the patient," but also one where the objective was to diagnose, provide a prognosis, and establish treatment (Martínez Cortés 2007, 197, my translation).

Several factors combined at this time to give rise to modern medicine in Mexico. Medicine was no longer considered to be separate from surgery; instead the two fields merged into the degree of *médico-cirujano* (physician-surgeon), a term still in use at the majority of Mexican medical schools today. French concepts about physiology were incorporated as central tenets of the curriculum (whereby bodies were understood in both their pathological and their normal states). And clinical approaches to medicine, particularly anatomy and pathology, became the primary ways to understand the body (Rodríguez 2008). By 1900, Mexico had nine medical schools, most of which were located in Mexico City (de la Garza-Aguilar 2005). This number increased exponentially during the twentieth century; by 2020, there were more than a hundred medical schools nationwide.[11]

MEDICINE IN PUEBLA

As I discussed in the introduction, Puebla is a large city. It was established during the sixteenth century and rapidly grew over the next few centuries to become the industrial city it is today. A city of contrasts, its race/color- and class-based hierarchy historically is visible in the distribution of populations into neighborhoods and in access to resources (Ramos 2012). Puebla looks toward the outside: it has attracted large car manufacturing plants like Audi and Volkswagen, a staggering array of global stores and brands, and thousands of tourists visiting its churches, monuments, museums, pyramids, and restaurants. Yet simultaneously it is very proudly insular, conservative, and *poblano*—to be descended from the Spanish colonizers, conveniently forgetting Puebla's origins of cultural and biological *mestizaje* (Cruz Bárcenas 2015).[12]

Hospitals were constructed as a priority in colonial Puebla. One of the first and largest hospitals was Hospital de San Pedro Apóstol, built in 1544, which functioned for almost 400 years (Fajardo-Ortíz 1999). It became the main space for learning medicine in Puebla, and by 1824 it housed the city's first formal medical school—the Medico-Surgical Academy of Puebla de los Ángeles. This institution countered the hegemonic pull of Mexico City, providing medical training to students whose modest social and economic backgrounds prevented them from migrating outside of Puebla (Castro Morales 2009, 4).

As elsewhere in Mexico, medicine in Puebla in the late nineteenth century was influenced by political and social forces, shaped by European scientific paradigmatic shifts about what medicine *was* and how it was to be practiced. Epidemics (smallpox, cholera, and typhus) were rampant, claiming thousands of lives (Agostoni 2003; Ramírez 2012). During the 1833 cholera epidemic in Puebla, there were only twenty-six physicians to attend to the 40,000 inhabitants; approximately 10 percent of the city's population died within five months (Malvido and Cuenya Mateos 2009). Informed by global concerns, the recurrent epidemics raised anxieties about social hygiene, sanitary reform, and hygiene education. The medical gaze moved from hospitals to public spaces, as new sites for managing health opened up.

Social hygiene, social control, and medicine have been heavily intertwined throughout Mexican history. The harsh colonial rule enacted upon Indigenous populations and the ensuing conflicts in the first few centuries after contact played a significant part in shaping people's health. Historian Paul Ramírez (2012, 231) states that although "disease was one of the great problems that animated intellectuals and reformers," the effects were most greatly felt by ordinary and nonliterate laypeople and so were of limited concern to those in power. The late nineteenth century began the process of solidifying bureaucracy into a system of population measurement and surveillance, drawing from science and scientific methods.

Such surveillance included medical enumeration and statistics, as well as eugenics and the reshaping of Mexican racial categories (Stern 1999; Secretaría de Salud 2017). Research focused on connecting morality, female hygiene, race, and nationalism, such as Francisco Flores y Troncoso's 1885 study on "The Mexican Hymen" or his 1888 study of women's pelvises where he concluded that Indigenous women's "backwards" anatomies would degenerate the nation (O'Brien 2013).[13] Studies such as these that incorporated racial science into obstetrics were emblematic of the nation's colonial and male concerns with control of women's bodies (Ruiz 2001), and they provide insight into matters of gender, class, and racialization. Because "history is never absent from . . . stories of racialized reproduction" (Rapp 2019, 729), the government was concerned with "problem" populations (prostitutes, Indigenous, the indigent) and concerns about *which* populations were reproducing (Braff 2013). By the early twentieth century moral hygiene was used as means of social control and as an explanation for the profound economic disparities and starkly unequal distribution of wealth. The emphasis on moralizing hygiene was a means to "condition conduct and to control society" (Rodríguez de Romo and Rodríguez Pérez 1998, 298, my translation).

A clear transition of medical care into state-level medicine was evident, whereby public health transformed into a key subject of governance and what

Agostoni (2007) calls an "unbreakable element of the nation's moral and material progress" (247, my translation). Between 1880 and 1915, Puebla saw an increase in educational and social welfare programs and infrastructure, including schools, universities, and trade schools as well as orphanages, mental health hospitals, and jails (Robles Galindo 2012). Many of these institutions were remodeled and standardized to mimic European concepts of human development and modernity, inscribing broader biopolitical ideals on institutional spaces and on the bodies of the populations. By the twentieth century, the previous European influence on Mexican medicine was replaced by the adoption of an American system of medicine, while also incorporating Mexican approaches with policies that emphasized disease prevention through poverty eradication and public health (Vaughn 2000; Finkler 2004).

At this time many hospitals, such as Hospital Piedad, were built (figure 7). Piedad was founded as a maternity hospital in 1885, when it was considered to be one of the largest hospitals for this purpose in Latin America. Some of the few written academic sources on the hospital state that its founder, a wealthy industrialist and philanthropist from an old poblano family, built the hospital as a haven for indigent women and single mothers (Sánchez Hernández and Dorel-Ferré 2008). The unofficial story, discussed in sources and told to me by one of the hospital directors, was that one day a man saw "a woman giving birth in a ditch and was deeply affected." This origin story interweaves class/race/color and gender as the founding principles of the hospital, which this philanthropist subsequently used to create a hospital foundation that carried his name so "women like her" could receive good maternity care. The Foundation continues to exist within the hospital, providing care to low-income and welfare populations, though it has become a subset of the larger hospital complex that caters to paying and insured patients.[14]

HOSPITAL SPACES AS HOSTILE SPACES

Gender inheres in female and male bodies, which can explain the gendered perceptions of aptitude and ability I described at the beginning of the chapter and how these have been internalized by both men and women. As Cassell (2000) states, the body (its size, manner, color, bearing, shape, etc.) expresses and reinforces social divisions between people. Some bodies are perceived to belong in certain spaces; others are out of place. The hostility or bias against women can be explained by the fact that women's bodies are not considered to belong in medical spaces, any more than they are thought to belong in fraternities or male clubs (Cassell 2000). Cassell (1997) argues that sacred spaces and their practices lose their potency if women are invited and learn their mysteries.

This gendered spatiality is seen in multiple ways, but it is perhaps best exemplified by the intersection of female gender, white uniforms, menstruation, and

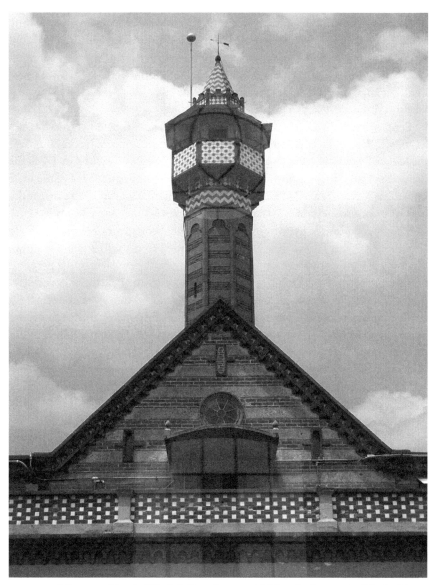

FIGURE 7. Minaret at Hospital Piedad. One doctor said, "People always ask if the building is strong. I show them the tower. [It] was built almost 150 years ago. And it is still there."

bathroom infrastructure. The standard uniform for the medical interns (and most residents) outside of the surgery wards was white in color. Scrubs could be any color or design the wearer chose, and they were often used as a canvas to express one's personality—like the interns who wore Winnie-the-Pooh or butterfly design scrubs or the obstetrician whose scrubs had an image of Taz from the Looney Tunes. One female resident in Hospital Salud would wear her white pants under bright pink scrubs; when she had to exit the sterile zone, she would strip off the scrubs like a superhero. Uniforms that were shabby were sources of criticism or jokes. Fourth-year resident Doctor Enrique teased third-year resident Doctora Valentina that "you cannot come into [this procedure] with that uniform" because it was so torn and patched.

People justified wearing the white uniforms because they portrayed doctors as "tidy," "clean," and "disciplined," because on a white uniform "stains are more evident and so the doctor always has to be clean" (see also Salhi 2016). Interns were penalized if their uniforms were scruffy, dirty, or incorrect. One of the male attending doctors at Piedad complained to me that the interns did not wear the correct uniform and that it "wasn't clean," that the women were not tying back their hair (required for hygiene), and that the men wore their ties as if they were "in a *cantina*" (bar). One intern, Amanda, tended to get into trouble with the doctors for various reasons. An intern with long curly black hair and a perpetually exhausted affect, she often spoke about balancing medical training with caring for her toddler as a single mother. When she wore white sweatpants instead of the requisite white trousers of the uniform, one of the hospital's directors gave her an official warning about her unprofessional behavior and for not following the hospital's rules. He explained to me that "if they're students, they have to wear the uniform, and their uniform is white." The only concession was the opportunity to wear scrubs during an overnight shift when they might engage "in activities that are very physically exhausting."

For women, wearing white during menstruation can be particularly inconvenient. Female trainees took extra precautions to make sure that they did not bleed through and stain their white clothes during their long hours on hospital rotations. Added to this was the reality that in many public hospitals in Mexico the bathrooms lack basic amenities like toilet seats, toilet paper, or strong water pressure. On many occasions over the years of fieldwork in public hospitals I witnessed how, by the end of the shift, the women's toilets were often grimy or clogged with paper and human waste, hampering people's ability to use them.

For some female interns, this lack of amenities added a layer of concern. This issue is marked by an "absent presence"—where spaces are designed for men and not for women, creating a gender data gap (Criado-Perez 2019). Diana was a lively intern from Hospital Piedad with light skin and hair, who took great care of her appearance. She sometimes struggled with the rigors of medicine. Although she had dreamed of other careers, she was pressured by her father to enter medicine because he believed it would provide her with better financial and job security. As she explained, "In the case of [medicine], it's harder [to be a woman]. From putting up with uncomfortable comments from a [male] doctor who is older than you are, to those aspects that have to do with hygiene." With a chuckle she added, "which a man does not [have], because of their anatomy; they don't have that type of infections like a woman does." She and other female interns mentioned that the inability to bathe would be physically uncomfortable for them in ways that men might not experience. Samantha, another intern at Piedad, did a short external rotation at a public hospital, and noted, "Here you're used to showering in the mornings. . . . And there I couldn't bathe, and so it was sometimes very uncomfortable." Diana added, "Yes, it's a profession that is still very, how would you say it, hostile to women." She concluded by illustrating how women's medical self was different than men's: "One really has to be very hard and mature [*dura y madura*] to manage it and know how to become skilled without getting burned [*saber desenvolverte sin quemarte*]."

Many of the issues I have described have to do with what Susan Hinze (1999) refers to as hierarchy of prestige—which is connected, quite literally, to practitioners' body parts—in what they can do and the metaphorical ways they are spoken about. Medicine is an institution clearly demarcated by male and female bodies and the symbolic ways they are enacted in these spaces. In many hospital spaces, female doctors are tokens; as sole representatives of their identity (Cassell 1997), they are often noticeably visible and have to work twice as hard and perform their work perfectly. This stress of perfection might lead them to react more sharply to errors in protocol, seeming to be "hysterical" or "tyrannical." These body parts are not gender neutral but rather carry significant gendered connotations. As Hinze (1999) argues, to "have balls" is to be tough, macho, and located higher on the hierarchy of prestige. Acting as metonyms, an association is established between men and these images of power (Cornwall and Lindisfarne 1994). As Hinze illustrates, the hierarchical structure of medicine places the masculine at the top (aggressive, active, macho) and the female (passive, affective, less physical) at the bottom *regardless of whether male or female bodies occupy these practices or spaces.*

This hierarchy is evident when people spoke about the different specialties and their gendered nature, speaking dismissively of those more suited to people who are more delicate and less strong. A specialty such as surgery is at the top of the medical hierarchy because it is an active specialty: hands probe, touch, fix, cut, and enter the body of patients, and practitioners (male or female) have "balls"—they are fearless in their practice and can endure the rigors of practice. By touching that which is hidden—for example, touching a uterus inside a woman's body—practitioners gain prestige. Drawing from Cassell's work (2000) Hinze states that the more embodied specialties carry the most prestige—that is, the bodies that are most active (such as orthopedic surgery) will carry greater prestige than those considered to be less active (such as dermatology, pediatrics, or psychiatry). The latter is always seen to be less macho, more feminine. When women become part of these spaces, the value system and the mental models (defined by men) do not necessarily change. Instead, women have to adapt and conform to these norms if they want to "belong." The spaces become "silent organizers" of mental and discursive maps people construct and inhabit (Hinze 1999, 234) as the female interns develop a medical self.

The white uniforms, combined with the poor bathrooms and infrastructure in some hospitals, have a much greater impact on women's bodies, cleanliness, and appearance, in many ways signaling that their bodies simply must adjust to the structure already in place that privileges male (non-menstruating) bodies. These are hostile spaces. Nicoletta Setola and colleagues (2013) show that the spatial configuration of a hospital can influence relationships and interactions between different people. In hospital training, I suggest, the hostile spaces that Diana has described also become toxic geographies (Mahtani 2014, 360); that is, the space itself is set up to privilege one group over another, creating a potentially poisonous environment where women's bodies do not fit. In order to fit, women sometimes must engage in what I term "dirty trade."

HARASSMENT AND HIERARCHY: "I'M USED TO DOCTORS SAYING *PENDEJADAS*"

Samantha's gamine appearance, pixie haircut, petite stature, and mischievous gaze belied a core of steel. She entered medicine because, when she was younger, her cousin had had an accident and received plastic and reconstructive surgery; the positive outcome made Samantha realize she wanted to be able to do that for other people. Intent on becoming a surgeon, she was aware of the macho attitude of many male doctors, especially as she was often a target of their comments. She recounted some of her experiences of being a woman in the medical field as we sat drinking coffee in the cafeteria of Hospital Piedad.

The cafeteria had only six tables and was set up on one corner of the hospital, open to the corridors. As we sat with our *lechero* coffees, I could see doctors, nurses, and patients walking by. The television on the wall loudly played variety shows, news, or 1980s music; the noise was sometimes drowned out by the whirring of blenders or espresso machines from the kitchen. Samantha shared how she handled the machismo and sexual harassment in a laparoscopic surgery she had been invited to watch a few months before. During the surgery the senior male surgeon spent much of the time harassing her, trying to rattle her. "I only went into surgery once with him and, after that, no more. . . . I went into surgery with him and his ego." She said that soon after the surgery began, he persisted in asking impertinent questions about whether she had been in his class at the university. When she curtly responded that she had not been in his class, he responded sourly, "Well, that's a shame, because otherwise you would now know a lot about anatomy."

Though on the surface this query about her training and knowledge about anatomy seems innocuous—after all, they were in a surgery where the knowledge of Anatomy (with a capital *A*) would be important information to have. Besides, she was an intern, and so her job was to learn. But Samantha recounted how the doctor shifted his commentary from describing the surgical procedures to descriptions of anatomy (with a lowercase *a*)—that is, anatomy as related to sexual intercourse. "He began to make comments to the [male] anesthesiologist. . . . I had only known the anesthesiologist for a little while. . . . And they began to comment stuff about sex and such." She added that she tried to intently focus on the laparoscopic surgery so she could tune out these comments, "so I was watching how things were going on the screen."

The surgeon, noticing her attention was not on him, commented, "Ay, poor *Doctorcita* [little female doctor], she has to hear all these things." Samantha replied, "Don't worry, Doctor, I'm used to it." She said she continued watching the screen, adding that the doctor asked her, nonplussed, "What are you used to? Sex?" She added that he said several more things that made her uncomfortable. So, she finally told him, "No, I'm used to [male] doctors saying *pendejadas* [bullshit] in the operating room."

Both of us laughed at this, each of us knowing just how much all the interns put up with, the female interns enduring the biggest share. Samantha concluded her story by saying that she did not speak a word to the physician during the rest of the surgery, adding with another chuckle, "I have never gone into [a procedure] with him again." She proudly said that after this the anesthesiologist always called her "La Respetada"—which loosely translates at the one who gained respect and owned the situation.

The interactions of many of the female participants with their male colleagues were what Iker, one of my male interlocutors at Hospital Salud, described as "tinged with sexual intent." He said, "My [female] friends here sometimes tell me with some fear and anxiety about the [suggestive] comments they've received. . . . [The men] take care not to say something really stupid, but they do insinuate, 'Let's go to this place,' or 'Let's go and do this thing,' or 'Okay, I'll accept the consult, but only because we're going out for coffee tomorrow.' Comments like that." His colleague Paola added, "Because I don't know what [men's] intentions are and I have no intention of doing anything. . . . I feel like that is where women suffer a bit more than men." Julieta from Hospital Piedad emphasized that interactions between men were different because "with a man it's more about friendship and they can rag on each other, with swear words, and so on." The culture of sexism in these spaces consisted of these forms of insinuations as well as comments on clothing, asking women to do the "female" work of typing or fetching coffee, or suggesting that women would not be able to cope with the rigors of training. Women felt that they had to "look out" for male doctors who were "interested in other things," who sat "really close and say inappropriate stuff," who wanted "to take advantage," or who wanted to "invite them out, to want that kind of stuff."

Many women in professional spaces experience microaggressions and overt discrimination and discouragement (Bhagwati 2019; Clancy et al. 2014; Lynn,

Howells, and Stein 2018). They have to deliberately work on not being too "girlie" in their dress, appearance (like painted nails), and mannerisms so they can "assume the characteristics" of the profession (Barthelemy, McCormick, and Henderson 2016). The explicit requests from attending doctors for women to tie back their hair and wear modest jewelry structurally shape how the women are meant to look and behave. Women might feel the need to mask their femininity through dress and demeanor, "muting" their observations on gender interactions, denying the harassment, and acting as "conceptual men" (Demaiter and Adams 2009:35). The female doctors I met in Mexico did not always act as conceptual men; instead they interwove their professional appearance—the white clothes and tied-back hair—with cultural perceptions of female beauty, which consisted of very detailed makeup routines and the use of feminine accessories like matching jewelry in their appearance.

Every morning at 7:00 A.M. the interns at Hospital Piedad met to hand over the night's cases to the day shifts. Most interns would arrive with wet hair from their shower. During this meeting, many of the female interns would use their time before the day's activity to apply makeup, extracting foundation, eyeliner, eye shadow, eyelash curlers, blush, and lipstick from their makeup bags while they discussed cases. They were expected to maintain their femininity. However, in a contradictory manner, because of the process of culturally stereotyping surgery as male, women with makeup and long nails are told that they do not fit (Riska and Novelskaite 2008) because their makeup and nail polish are classified as unhygienic and foci of infection. Because appearance was one of the first (and most easily policed) steps in developing a medical self, women had to balance these expectations about general medical appearance (professional, clean, organized) with the expectations of a feminine appearance (jewelry, makeup) as they developed their medical self.

One of Iker's closest friends at Hospital Salud was Rosa, a reserved and well-liked intern whose shyness seemed to embolden others to harass her. She had attended the public medical school in Puebla because the education was free, and she chose this hospital for her internship because her parents were patients in the public health-care system and she had seen the good care they received. We talked over coffee about her experiences and labors as an intern, and how she managed the time constraints, the lack of sleep, the overwork, and learning many new skills. She said, "At first I could not *aguantar* [endure] them. I think that in my first three or four months I cried a lot. I actually wanted to leave [medicine]." She added that she often felt uncomfortable with the male residents. She said that many times "we're writing up notes and they sit really close to us, and they start to invite you to go on a date, or to go to the movies. . . . So it's like an uncomfortable feeling. Or they make jokes in poor taste."

On one occasion I observed Rosa at the nurses' station in obstetrics filling out medical charts. The nurses' station was against one wall facing four patient beds draped in pink and white sheets. Behind the nurses' station was a cabinet with medications. On a high ledge above a table with blankets was a small altar that consisted of a small wooden house sitting on a lace cloth, with a golden cross drawn on it and a small pot with fake flowers inside. A small blue toy car incongruously sat next to the altar. When Rosa finished the charts, she handed them to Doctor Enrique, the senior male obstetrics resident in the ward that day, who many of the women avoided. He was often abusive, and would curse at interns if they did not do the work correctly. As he took the papers from Rosa, he joked that she should write her name on them as "Rosa Salvaje" (wild rose).[15] Rosa did not smile, her tense shoulders indicating her dislike of the comment. In response to her silence and unsmiling countenance, Doctor Enrique patted her back in a familiar way. His tone and subsequent pat on the back illustrated the sexual intent to which Iker had referred. This was particularly evident with his use of the word "salvaje," which suggested that she was untamed or sexually adventurous. I could tell that Rosa was uncomfortable by both this interaction and the underlying assumptions about her sexuality. However, like many of her female peers, she just continued doing the work she was expected to do, enduring the harassment and comments. Most women said they felt ill equipped to address such harassment. Trainees internalize these disquieting, problematic, or "morally unsettling" (Hafferty and Franks 1994, 118) practices, ultimately accepting them as routine, ordinary, and just part of training.

All the female interns I met had experienced some form of harassment that had made them uncomfortable though most of them brushed it off as an inevitable part of being a smart and competent woman in a man's world. Uncomfortable interactions between men and women usually mapped onto hierarchy, like in Rosa's or Samantha's experiences where the harassers were residents or attending physicians. Women in these circumstances sometimes second-guessed their reactions to harassment while others placed blame on the female victims themselves for being "sensitive." Ironically, given the harassment she experienced with the surgeon's "pendejadas," Samantha told me that women are too sensitive: "It's a defect I see that some of the girls here have. They think that all the male doctors are flirting with them or want something more. . . . The [men] notice; they always notice. And so they continue with the game, and the [women] don't know how to reply to the [doctors], so the game doesn't become problematic."

Such beliefs reinforce these gendered norms, sexist behaviors, and an acceptance of the "totemic illusion" (Gutmann 2005, 84) of men's sexuality as naturalized and taken for granted, which equates "male sexuality with uncontrollable urges." This approach removes any form of blame on men's harassment, instead placing the onus of responsibility on women to deal with it. This fear of being "too sensitive" could prevent victims from seeking redress for the behaviors (Hinze 2004). They place the blame on themselves rather than on individuals' sexist behavior and the institutionalized sexism present in the hospital.

"I WANT A PRINCESS": THE DIRTY TRADE OF TRAINING

Although most female trainees internalized and accepted the harassment as ordinary in these spaces, Diana really struggled with it. Her experience with harassment can be considered to be extraordinary in many ways, but it is also deeply illustrative of the ways that it is engendered in training and how women experience various forms of violence in their lives. When we met in 2016, she was beginning the second half of her internship year at Hospital Piedad, but she had just transferred from another hospital because of experiences with pervasive harassment. In our conversations we spoke at length about issues of gender and medical training.

She described the immensely hard physical labor that was expected of interns at her former internship, where they pushed heavy gurneys, attended to dozens of patients without rest, and literally dashed across the night-darkened hospital campus for bloodwork and other laboratory tests. Almost anyone would be fearful of walking across a large hospital's courtyard in the dark, particularly one located in one of the more dangerous neighborhoods of the city; a woman can feel especially vulnerable in these circumstances. Believing that they were treated like cheap manual labor and like secretaries, she said she felt let down by medicine during her first semester as an intern; she began to feel depressed and ready to leave the program because of the hard work and the harassment.

> As a woman you have to put up with comments, threats, messages, whatever. And what it really affected was learning, because what you want to do is learn. So you arrive with the best attitude so that people want to teach you, and then most of the [men] confuse good attitude with flirting or something else, right? And so I would come up to a [male] doctor and ask, "Doctor, can you teach me to put on a splint?" [He would say], "Sure, but how about if we go out for a coffee before that?"

These forms of gendered transactional bargaining were not experienced by her male peers. Diana said that if men asked to learn a procedure the male physician would respond, "Yes, look, you put this here, and you move that there." She asked crossly, "So, like, why does it have to be different? [...] It's much harder [*pesado*] for a woman." Her use of the word "pesado" is interesting because its dual meaning can suggest harder but also heavier; its latter meaning was often used when describing women's inability to lift heavy limbs during surgery. I asked whether she was the only one at that hospital who was harassed. She replied, "No, I think there were more girls, but most don't dare to speak up about what is happening, and, well, I was the only one who complained." She added that women were silent about this "because of fear, because in fact, many of the [male] doctors threaten us, like, 'don't you say anything or I'll lower your grade.' So you prefer to *aguantar* [endure], and so you stay quiet."

Silence of this sort is quite common, as evidenced by Rosa's and Diana's stories. Few victims of harassment directly confront their harasser, and most agree that active resistance could be professionally devastating—through a loss of a job, poor performance reviews, or dismissal from a training program (Hinze 2004). Others feel that speaking out about inequities might jeopardize their careers in ways that those with privilege would not experience (Lynn, Howells, and Stein 2018) or even recognize as problematic.

I asked Diana whether she and her female peers ever spoke about these issues among themselves, given that they spent so much time together in the hospital. She said that in private the women would say, "Doctor *Fulano* [Dr. X] said this to me, and Doctor *Sutano* [Dr. Y] sent me this." She added that most of the women would say to each other, "It's only a year, so I just have to aguantar one year." But she said, with a chuckle, "No, I don't have to aguantar a year," adding that the situation was hard and that she was determined to leave, especially as she did not feel she was learning much at that hospital anyway. She said that if she had been learning a lot, then "it's worth it for me to aguantar." The verb aguantar is amply used in all sorts of contexts in Mexico; it is not limited to encounters within medicine. It is a common verb about enduring life in general.

Diana shared that the chief of clinical training (*Jefa de Enseñanza*) at that hospital was a woman. I asked her whether the chief's gender made her more empathetic about the harassment. Diana admitted that she never had the courage to tell her specifically about the harassment, but instead blamed the hard work conditions as her reason for wanting to transfer. Her choice to emphasize the work as the official reason for leaving unintentionally reinforced the idea pervasive in these hospital spaces that women do not have the fortitude for hard medicine or for enduring its difficulties and labor. It also silenced her voice and emboldened the perpetrators. A lack of endurance is also linked to perceptions of being delicadas and is likely also a contributing factor of sexual harassment. That is, if a woman is delicate (and weak), she is seen to be more pliable and less likely to notice harassment (or complain about it).

Diana also admitted that one of the reasons for not officially reporting the harassment was because she was threatened by the men who had harassed her. She said that they told her "if you tell the Doctora, I will do this." She added, "So it was hard for me." She later mentioned that when she first began the internship, the chief had specifically told the female trainees that if they ever faced any issues with harassment or lack of respect, they should tell her. Diana said that the chief encouraged the female interns to involve the necessary authorities rather than trying to address the issue on their own. The chief's words suggest that she might have been aware that there was gender-based harassment at the hospital and was aiming to create a mechanism for women to come forward. This effort to uncover gender issues is what Sara Ahmed (2012, 17) calls nonperformative; that is, an institution performs an image of itself where the performance of the good intention is the sole objective, rather than an effort to change the system. In doing so, "they do not bring about the effects they name." Diana laughed ruefully and said, "We know that in Mexico this always happens; I'm not sure if in other countries. It's a problem that exists, and it exists in all hospitals . . . for a long time and that doesn't change. I doubt it will ever change." Sighing, she said, "Although I didn't know [medicine] would be this hard. . . . So sometimes when I am very tired, or very stuck, or just *nefasteada* [fed up] with the day and such, I say, 'I should have been a chef.'"

The gendered organizational structure of these medical spaces structures perceptions about women, such as female vulnerability, beauty, or "female-like" skills. Elianne Riska and Aurelija Novelskaite (2008, 231), drawing from Erving Goffman's work (1959), referred to this as "gender casting," where tasks are a priori assigned with gender assumptions. For instance, women are assumed to be good at helping, being organized, or good at secretarial tasks, like Diana said in her narrative; men are assumed to be better suited for active duties like cutting and suturing, or are emotionally composed and stoic during surgery or when being scolded. Some doctors in these hospitals were known to treat women like "princesses"—not as colleagues but as delicate creatures who could not hear crudeness or deal with blood and other bodily fluids. They also generally treated the female interns with greater care than they did the men. Female interns learned to tolerate these male doctors or to come up with ways to deal with their behavior. As Cassell's (1997) work among female surgeons showed, gendered scripts in medicine are so deeply embedded that they occur unthinkingly and are unquestioned. Because so many of the practices, narratives, and beliefs that both male and female trainees heard and witnessed in these spaces subtly and not-so-subtly emphasized a gendered difference, most of my participants would accept these beliefs and practices as "naturally given."

In a profession such as medicine, women must learn the process of "doing gender." That is, women have to comply with and sustain masculine norms that celebrate a masculine vision (Bolton and Muzio 2008, 283), where the feminine is marginalized. Women are consequently often stereotyped into gendered roles (Cassell 1997), yet the female surgeons in Cassell's study did gender in different ways. She argued that men "did dominance" (as surgeons) and women "did deference" (as nurses). My female interlocutors were often gender cast into secretarial duties so they could "do deference." The women in Cassell's study who displayed agonistic or dominant behaviors were socially sanctioned. Women are taught to underplay their achievements, and to value humility; this underplaying might ultimately have effects on women's confidence in their skills and their identity as physicians (Blanch et al. 2008).

Some of my male interlocutors from both hospitals described their observations of gender relations in these spaces, like one who explained, "my *compañeras* [female workmates] told me that being a woman was an advantage in the internship because there are many male doctors [here, and] they can get along better, right? . . . There are doctors who are somewhat coy. . . . They like a woman to be in their ward because they are men. And, I don't know, maybe because of a visual thing or something." Another man said that some male attending physicians specifically requested women with words such as "No, I don't want him; I want a woman. I want a princess." In these spaces both referential and indexical markers of gender were present—wherein to be female or not possess "masculine" markers and behaviors (aggressiveness, arrogance) was to not entirely belong (Cornwall and Lindisfarne 1994). Even though they might have been invited into procedures, this invitation was a form of dirty trade—that is, women had to be "beautiful," docile, and humble to entice particular male physicians to extend an invitation into a procedure.

THE FIRM HAND OF MASCULINITY

Although these spaces tended to foster a more hegemonic masculinity, not all the men inhabiting them ascribed to this perception. One of the older physicians at Hospital Piedad, Doctor Contreras, candidly shared his own perceptions of masculinity. "Knowing [how to do housework] doesn't take away your masculinity. . . . But that's how we were brought up, not knowing how to fold a shirt, make a scrambled egg, or a *licuado* [smoothie]. . . . When did I learn to do these? During residency." As scholars of gender and masculinity have shown, masculinities emerge, change, and are part of a broader process, which at times might be contradictory and seemingly irreconcilable (Wentzell 2013). Emily Wentzell (2013, 26), in her ethnographic examination of men, aging, and illness in Mexico, suggested the concept of composite masculinity to understand "how individuals construct and revise their gendered selfhood across time and context" and as "contingent and fluid constellations of elements that men weave together into masculine selfhoods." Both she and other scholars of masculinity in Mexico (Brandes 2002; Gutmann 1996; Mirandé 2018) have shown how gender is a nuanced and context-contingent performance, wherein masculinity can be understood as what men say and do *to be men* (Gutmann 1996, 17, italics in original).

Bianca, from Hospital Salud, referenced what Cassell (1997) calls teaching by humiliation when she said, "[Male residents] feel that we are still the weaker sex, because they don't scold us the same as men. . . . [They] will yell at a man, swear at him, . . . but a woman, no. [The doctor] makes you see your mistakes, but he doesn't yell at you. . . . They do have a firmer hand [*mano dura*] with men."[16] A male intern at Hospital Piedad described how one male neurosurgeon who was known to be rude and aggressive toward men was much gentler with the women "because with men he has more liberty to swear at him and whatever he wants." One of my female interlocutors put it bluntly, "[The male doctors] prefer the girls a little bit more because they know that we will not answer back too much;

they will not have as many problems with us." Mano dura in training suggested a certain indulgence of a woman's "delicate nature" that was not extended to men, but the disparity in treatment seemed to benefit no one. When I asked what effect this had on learning, Bianca replied, "It is not beneficial because, I don't know, they should treat us all the same because then there are like conflicts between us, like, 'He did not yell at you because you're a girl' or, you know, 'he likes you.'"

One female intern added that some doctors "take it out on the guys [*se desquitan*]; so guys need to look out for those." Kevin, a very easygoing intern at Hospital Salud, referenced this type of interaction by saying, "When many of my *compañeros* are scolded, they feel bad. Here we call that '*se agüitan*' [they "water," i.e., cry]." He stated that most times these punishments were about the ego of people higher on the medical hierarchy who imposed their will on others. "Here they use their power based on the hierarchy; they feel that because they have a better [higher] rank they can do what they like to you, say what they want to you, punish you like they want, sometimes for very absurd things. . . . They tell you that this forms your character, forms you personally, and you should not take it as a scolding nor punishment but like a lesson." He believed however that one worked best in a harmonious environment where there was cooperation and empathy between everyone, rather than abuse and people's explosive outbursts of "this is my power, and I will make you feel bad."

What attributes of maleness are empowering in these spaces? What happens when someone is perceived to be "weaker" than expected? Men were the objects of mano dura training, and because of gendered norms of behavior they were expected to not complain. If they did complain, they would be considered unmasculine. As Kenneth Matos, Olivia O'Neill, and Xue Lei (2018) stated, in environments that are highly toxic, toxic leaders are not seen to be abnormal or out of place; instead, people who "do not fit" begin to have self-doubts about their own belonging and question their skills and abilities to thrive in that professional world.

Some of Iker's peers and supervisors tended to make fun of him because he did not quite "fit" in the culture of the ward and was perceived to not be as masculine as others. He was a gentle, introspective intern who spoke softly and did not fit the hegemonic masculinity definitions of successfully "being a man" (Cornwall and Lidisfarne 1994). In one interview I asked him to describe the various doctors and residents whom he had helped as an *instrumentista* [scrub technician]. He said that one of the most difficult residents to work with was Doctor Enrique, the fourth-year resident at Hospital Salud who harassed Rosa and who many interns avoided as much as possible. He said that when interns did not know something Doctor Enrique felt they should know, "he really scolds us, he throws [us out of the room], he hits us, he yanks things from us." I was surprised at some of the verbs he used and asked what he meant by "hit." Iker said that Doctor Enrique would rap them with the clamps. As he explained this, he motioned the act of rapping someone's knuckles ("pow"). He said that Doctor Enrique would tell interns that he yearned for the days when interns could be hit "to really make [them] bleed, . . . and would like to do the same to us as much as the law will allow." Iker then compared this doctor with others who would scold him appropriately "when they are meant to, and in the decibels that should be used," who would at times even tell him "you have done well."

Mano dura and harsher scolding for men also reflected the paternalism woven into the medical setting and broader gendered social norms, where, as Aarón from Hospital Piedad said, men would be naturally more courteous to female than to male interns. He explained that this disparity was acceptable because men were more able to tolerate mistreatment and verbal abuse while women were more likely to become stressed and upset: "And you're like, 'Damn! I'm scared of this doctor, but, oh well, I have to be there.'" He emphasized what he perceived to be men's natural stoicism and their ability to distance themselves personally from scolding and harsh language. And yet, as some studies have shown (Davis and Allison 2013), mistreatment in medical school significantly affects career decisions. Such a gendered form of training signals to everyone that men are stronger and better able to take brutal or harsh treatment. But the impact of this harshness can be significant on men's mental well-being and eventual medical forms of practice and teaching style.

By participating and working in these spaces, trainees develop a medical self that is nuanced, flexible, and fluid. It is shaped not only by the broader history of medicine but also by the particular ways of doing things in different spaces and what Joseph Calabrese (2011) refers to as the assumptions of medical institutions. Diana put it most succinctly when she said, "It's true that the upper hierarchy is always managed by men. So that influences the way that the hospital interacts with women. . . . The directors, who are men, are quite pleasant to women, and, like, they defend them and all that. But their authority is also lost at some point; from some point down [the hierarchy] just does what it wants, right?" These contingent medical selves, like the composite masculinities of the men of Wentzell's (2013) study, might seem to be inherently contradictory. That is, at times women might do deference, at others they are assertive, and in still others they learn to manage the system. By the same token, in some contexts the men might align with more hegemonic forms of masculinity, while in others they eschew these as abuse.

What does it mean to belong (or not) in medical spaces? How does (un)belonging shape one's practice and medical self? Subsequent chapters address these questions, and show how medical selving goes beyond Marcel Mauss's (1973) techniques of the body and Pierre Bourdieu's ([1977] 2000) habitus and is a deeper engagement between the body, practice, thoughts, and action, especially whether and how interns learn to employ their body as a means to understand and measure the world around them.

I WILL AGUANTAR

Female interns' experiences showcase the (extra)ordinary presence of women in hospital spaces, particularly how perceptions of female incompetence and weakness are interwoven with sexual innuendos, microaggressions, and misogyny. Women in these spaces learn to aguantar these encounters and persist toward their goal. Their "delicate" bodies as female doctors are always gendered (sexualized, eroticized, or excluded), remaining marked (Beagan 2000). Because the verb aguantar was used so frequently by my interlocutors to talk about endurance and abilities in medical practice, I have chosen to elaborate on its contextual meaning here.

The male and female interns' experiences provide a lot to think with, especially the multiple and gendered ways by which the verb aguantar is used. The men I interviewed primarily seemed to use the idea of endurance to talk about women's lack of strength and consequent inability to last in surgical procedures, in specific specialties, or even in medicine as a whole. That is, men have "balls" (Hinze 2004), are fearless in their practice, and can aguantar anything. The way that Diana uses endurance flips this concept on its head. She and the other women whose stories she shared used aguantar to describe the ability to persist through hardship and to endure a hostile or problematic work environment in order to achieve one's goals, in turn developing a determined medical self, able to manage these unfolding scenarios, embodying more toughness and resistance. Notably, endurance as used by the women requires no change in the system—not on the part of the person having to endure, nor in the person creating the situation that needs endurance, nor in structures that force one's endurance. Instead aguantar for the women is about accepting the reality of gendered violence, finding the strength to continue, and persisting in one's efforts to succeed. Female interns were deliberate in the ways they interacted, walking a fine line between being too eager, too hard working, too pliable or feminine, and too competent. If they simply acted "as women" without any of this deliberate cultivation they would not gain entrance into the more male-guarded sphere of surgical and other procedures.

The stories of Samantha, Rosa, and Diana illustrate the multiple intersecting forms of vulnerability that female trainees embody, and yet they also show how this powerlessness can be used against those in power. These women were vulnerable in several ways: as interns they were at the bottom of the medical hierarchy; as women they were stereotyped as being too emotional, delicate, or weak; and as youths they could be treated with less respect by the older physicians and thus harassed. All these forms of harassment should have been extraordinary, though because of their ubiquity they were quite ordinary in these spaces. All three interns were vulnerable in those contexts because each was part of a hospital structure managed by men who were older and had the power to affect the women's positions in the internship by reporting them to hospital directors. This vulnerability probably explains why for the most part they, and other female interns like them, silently endured so much criticism and harassment from their superiors and why Samantha's retort to the surgeon's "pendejadas" was so particularly powerful.

My interlocutors' experiences illustrate the underlying and unidirectional tension between male physicians and female interns. There was an enactment of power and authority in these interactions, within which the idea of young female pliability was also enmeshed. While these interactions were not always exploitative, they did tend to follow lines of hierarchy: that is, an older male physician or resident harasses a younger female intern (or junior resident). This overt form of discrimination arises from underlying, hidden structures that continue to discriminate against those who "do not belong." These interactions and structures are ordinary and normative, though they should be rare. The underlying structures are a much subtler form of harassment and discrimination, which might use practices such as double standards, discouragement, biased referral patterns, or gendered funding patterns (Bruce et al. 2015) that dissuade women from persisting. The culturally produced message that many women receive early in medical training is that women are different (Riska and Novelskaite 2008).

Judith Butler (1993) has argued that the construction of gender is active and quasi penetrative, with gender emerging by absorbing and displacing sex. This form of gender construction is divinely performative, "bringing into being and exhaustively constituting that which it names" (1993, 6). Because "female" is considered out of place in hospital professional spaces, female interns are not "properly gendered" (Butler 1993). Hence, women have to constantly perform and reinterpret their belonging, and shift from extraordinary to ordinary—through their clothing, makeup, language, efforts to aguantar and fight against perceptions of being delicadas, or even their very presence in these spaces. "Race, class, and gender," Cassell argues, "inhere in bodies, tangible bodies as well as 'imaginary bodies'—those images, symbols, and beliefs that shape social and political reality for individuals and groups" (2000, 48). Bodies are thus indistinguishable from the norms that govern their materiality (Butler 1993). Women have to perform the role of "woman doctor"—a dynamic identity that represents female medical students' reconciliation of their identities of women and medical trainees, which is constantly informed and shaped by institutional culture and stereotyped gender roles (Babaria et al. 2012, 1014).

Rosa said, with a rueful laugh, "Over time I think that one starts to get used to the scoldings, to cry when you are meant to cry, and just study. I think that's how I am aguantando right now. If I have to cry, I do it, and then I do other things so I forget about it." Like Butler, I believe that this process of coping with harassment and performing a certain gendered identity as woman doctor is not a singular "act," but rather is reiterative and deliberate (1993, 2) as part of a process of reminding themselves and their peers and mentors that they belong and are there to stay, and as part of the deeper process of creating a gendered medical self. Because of all these structures, most of the female medical students and interns I met experienced a dual form of learning: they not only learned the skills and techniques, like any other medical student, but they also learned how to navigate gender dynamics to stay safe and actually learn, even though this process could be exhausting.

2 · DOCTORS ON THE MARCH
Punishment, Violence, and Protests

I believe in a socialist medicine.... We should all have access to health because it's not a privilege; it's not something that you earn; it's something that you deserve as a right, and it's shameful that not everyone has [access].
—Kevin, intern at Hospital Salud

I think that what most bothers me about medicine is that there are people who can't pay for it. —Amanda, intern at Hospital Piedad

It's kind of the culture, right? Like, "because you are a medical intern, I'm going to treat you badly," and the attending physician is going to treat the resident badly, and the resident treats the intern [that way], like that. Because you're the one on the lowest rung, it's always, like, "go for the paper and do this, and you can't sleep in this bed, and go for that."
—Julieta, intern at Hospital Piedad

Two days after the bus accident I was still exhausted from staying up all night. I slept in longer than usual and arrived at Hospital Piedad by late morning. When I met the interns, they excitedly greeted me with "You're late! You missed a code red." One intern gleefully said that the code was fantastic, even though the patient, an elderly woman, had died. The patient had started coding while interns Mauricio and Emilio were on the hospital ward, although they first thought her machine had simply become unplugged. But when they went into her room and checked her with their stethoscope, they realized she had no heartbeat. Both interns then began cardiopulmonary resuscitation (CPR), and were joined by an emergency room (ER) physician, but with no success. The patient died. Seemingly unconcerned about the outcome of the code, the interns' excitement about the experience was evident, as they laughed and joked that now they knew where their gaps in knowledge were. Emilio, a confident intern who tended to take the lead among his peers, turned to another intern who often fell asleep during meetings and had acquired the reputation for being less knowledgeable than the others, and joked that even he could now run a "*clasesita*," a little class, on code reds and CPR. This intern turned to me and said in a mock hurt voice, surrounded by the laughter of his peers, "Have you written this down in your notebook? See how they treat me?"

Though I understood their gallows humor in response to tragedy, from my outsider's perspective I found it hard to reconcile their excitement with the grim reality of a patient dying on their watch. Physician Damon Tweedy (2015) refers to the glee felt by doctors as the "soap opera element" that, in these spaces, passes for normal behavior. What is important to note is that these behaviors happened backstage—away from the patients and other doctors—where the interns could shed some of the trappings of performing their public medical self (Goffman 1959).[1] When trainees were frontstage, they were expected to perform their medical self before their superiors, the nurses, the patients, and the patients' families (Good 1995a). This performance was sometimes low stakes, where they simply acted like doctors through dress and manner, which, as Mary-Jo DelVecchio Good (1995a) has suggested, sometimes gets muddled with actual competence. But sometimes, such as when a patient coded, the stakes were much higher, and their performance included actual medical and life-saving skills—which sometimes failed. Trainees negotiated a tight balance between competence and caring (Carpenter-Song 2011), where competence was associated with more overt skills, knowledge, or use of technical language while caring was more about interpersonal skills, attitude, compassion, or empathy (Good and Good 1989). The gallows humor became a way for them to cope with tragedy.

In thinking through the juxtaposition of their heightened emotions and the reality of death, I remembered a conversation I had had with Amanda some days before about another patient death. She described how in her very first *guardia* (overnight shift) as an intern, a patient had died after colon surgery and that the whole ward smelled strongly of intestinal decay and death. Shuddering, she said that the death, combined with the foul odor, stayed with her for days. She said she was still very spooked and that she "felt weird . . . when we get patients who could be possible code reds. . . . I feel like they could die any minute if we're not careful or something." As one scholar has noted, "Medicine is an odd profession, in which we ask ordinary people to act as if feces and vomit do not smell, unusual bodies are not at all remarkable, and death is not frightening" (Watson 2011, 43).

Later that morning I walked with Aarón to the ER. He was a very tall and thin intern who entered medicine at the urging of his father, and he had acquired a quiet confidence in his abilities. His peers described him as someone who was always in a good mood and unfazed by stressful situations. We passed by the family of the deceased patient congregated in the lounge just outside the ER's double doors. They sat on the black couches in small groups, looking worn with grief. Some held each other and cried; others had tear-stained faces and red eyes. Their grief tugged at me, heightening my feeling of awkwardness in these spaces. Aarón commented *soto voce* that the patient had been older and was already sick with nephropathy and systemic edema (kidney failure and swelling). She had been in intermediate care, but he wondered whether she should instead have been in the intensive care unit (ICU). His tone, while low, did not convey concern about the death itself but more of an acceptance that the situation was out of their hands. Everyone who works with people who are sick has crossed "the boundary into the space where human mortality and finitude—and the feelings of helplessness associated with them—come to the fore" (Piemonte 2015, 388).

In the ER some of the interns were taking a short break between patients. The ER had eight curtained cubicles and a small staff to attend the patients who came for treatment for minor emergencies—mostly broken bones, falls, and some car crashes. Most of their patients were children because the hospital had contracts with several local schools. They attended approximately sixty patients daily. The large nurses' station stood between the cubicles and the ambulance entrance, which indicated its important position in the space. It was both a central work-space where clinicians filled out forms and looked at medical records and a central gathering place for socializing when the ward was emptier.

Today the interns stood at the nurses' station chatting with Doctora Rocío Duarte, an ICU physician. She was feared by most of the interns and was known for her sharp criticism of shoddy practice and of frequently banishing from the ICU trainees who did not work to her standards. On that day, likely prompted by the death of the patient, she was giving the interns advice on the need to develop non-medical skills and to protect themselves from legal troubles. Dressed in black pants and brown blouse, with a chic leather jacket and short, bobbed brown hair, she looked like she was about to exit the hospital rather than being in the middle of her work day. She cautioned the interns, "You have to be very methodical. You have to learn to legally defend yourselves," reminding them that they should write all the medical notes correctly and carefully "or you'll never stand a chance" against being sued. She added that the *Ministerio Público* (the national jurisprudence and prosecutorial ministry) does not distinguish between interns and senior physicians, so their junior rank would not protect them against legal action. Doctora Duarte told them that they needed to become used to doing things correctly and that they should request that the hospital provide them with a legal protection learning module, emphasizing her suspicion of patients and the legal system, "*Cuídense* [be careful]; trust no one."

Her dire warning was followed by a description of her own legal disputes. Doctora Duarte said, "Something that took me sixteen years to learn is conscientious objection." She explained that, hypothetically, they might one day have a patient whose medical condition they identified after a lengthy process of running all the necessary tests and consulting with other hospital physicians; yet the patient's family might refuse treatment. She said that if that happened, as doctors they needed to write down in the medical notes that treatment was refused by the family. She told them that they should subsequently recuse themselves from the case and write "conscientious objection" on the notes. She said, "I've had it up to *here*," revealing that she had had three suits filed against her.

A couple of months before, Doctora Duarte and César, a hard-working but anxious intern, co-presented a case about a female patient at a weekly *caso clínico* (grand rounds). The patient was obese with chronic abnormal menstrual bleeding and high cholesterol, who arrived at 11:00 P.M. on December 31 at the ER experiencing severe shortness of breath and vomiting. An examination showed a large mass in her uterus and an infection ("she had everything"). A clinical history revealed that she had been at the beach in Acapulco three days before where she had scuba-dived; she then spent over three hours driving back up the mountains to Puebla, when she began to feel unwell. The doctors considered that she had either acute coronary syndrome or pulmonary thrombosis. Doctora Duarte said, "Honestly, the family members were very stubborn. Even though we explained it to them, they didn't understand [the severity]. . . . That type of patient *must* be in the ICU, okay? [. . .] We finally proposed to put in a vena cava filter (placed in the leg vein to prevent clots from moving to the lungs). But her husband considered that we were exaggerating and that she didn't have anything, so he requested a voluntary discharge. And she went home, without oxygen, because he said that God would cure her." They never knew the patient's outcome.

Doctors often had horror stories to tell the interns. In these clinical narratives, physicians played a nodal part (directing the action, the treatment, the course of the disease, etc.), but social and institutional forces outside their control (like the request from a patient's family) can disrupt or fragment the story (Good 1995b, 464). In this narrative doctors tended to portray themselves as a moral medical self, as when an otorhinolaryngology surgeon told the interns during another session that death was not always the doctor's fault: "It depends on one's experience, it depends on the surgeon."[2] He described a former patient with poorly managed diabetes who died the day after surgery at one of the public hospitals. He said it happened because the hospital had too many patients and not enough residents over the weekend, and an intern improperly performed a procedure. Emphasizing concerns with legal issues and echoing Doctora Duarte's warning about trusting no one, he concluded by encouraging the interns to find their moral professional voice (Good 1995a): "If a patient dies it is a risk; it is a professional risk because you can be sued even if it's not your fault."

The doctors often emphasized caution with using terms such as sentinel event (an unanticipated event resulting in death or harm). During a clinical case at Hospital Salud, a neonatal ICU doctor described a baby born with gastroschisis (where the bowel develops outside of their body). He said, "No one committed the defect or sepsis, which, though we can think of them as quasi-faults or adverse events, they are not brought about by a medical system. Here medical error is not considered. . . . It is something congenital that we cannot change."

Because it was a slow day with few patients, Doctora Duarte's conversation with the interns drew in some of the senior doctors on duty, who began to trade stories about legal issues faced by other doctors they knew: a doctor at a public hospital accused of murder because he treated a patient who did not disclose her hemophilia and bled out; a doctor accused of sexual abuse after his patient undressed without waiting for a nurse to be in the room. To the listening clinicians, these stories underscored their prevailing belief that doctors followed the moral behavior of doing everything possible for a patient (Bosk 2003). Yet these stories highlighted a tension between the personhood of patients, as a "construct of jural rights and moral accountability" (Scheper-Hughes and Lock 1987, 14), and their own medical rights that were often limited by their patients' rights. These stories also served to organize and interpret their medical experiences, create idealized ways of interacting with patients, and "[formulate] reality and idealized ways of interacting with it" (Good 1994, 80). In the process they might forget that their practice is based on the principle of serving others and doing no harm (Casas-Patiño et al. 2013).

Doctora Duarte cautioned the interns, especially the men, that they should protect themselves and always attend female patients with a nurse in the room. She emphasized that they should never go into a patient's room alone or they could be accused of rape, and that would be the end of their career. She concluded by saying, "In these things, the woman has more strength than the man." Before she could elaborate on this perspective, her cellphone rang with a call from the ICU. She listened to the person on the other end, nodded a few times, and hung up. She said, "I made a mistake with a medicine." As she walked to the elevators, she told the interns that one of her patients was *desaturando* (exhibiting hypoxia, low concentration of oxygen in arterial blood) and that she had to go.

In this chapter I examine the paradoxical tussle between doctors as simultaneously powerful and powerless by returning to the broader political economic structure of the country and examining how this shapes doctors' abilities to practice and how it both imbues them with the power over patients' lives and strips them of their ability to withstand abuses from the broader system. Sometimes patients die; sometimes doctors make tragic mistakes; sometimes doctors are demonized for these deaths; and sometimes these deaths are caused by factors outside of doctors' control. The ordinary practice of medicine is punctuated by extraordinary moments that can bring medical selves into sharp relief. These dueling forces of external and internal, ordinary and extraordinary deeply shape doctors' sense of self. Trainees learn that they can be powerful doctors but can also be victims of abuse and of structures that demonize and disregard them.

I draw from the work of Mexican sociologist Roberto Castro, who has explored medical training and the violence surrounding medicine. His recent work with

Marcia Villanueva Lozano (2018) highlights the juxtaposition between external violence (such as legal cases with judiciary ministries, state-level policies affecting health care, and doctors being victims of narco-violence) and the violence internal to the medical spaces (violence toward patients or violence between clinicians). Castro and Villanueva Lozano argue that physicians are outspoken against the former because they see external violence affecting their bodily integrity, their professional identity, or their ability to practice. This criticism is evident in Doctora Duarte's admonishments to the interns to protect themselves from crafty patients or lawyers. However, doctors are often blind to internal forms of violence (Castro and Villanueva Lozano 2018) because the symbolic, physical, or emotional violence enacted in hospital spaces is seen as natural and as part of transforming into a doctor. It is a process of unseeing the violence. I showcase the paradoxes of my interlocutors' practice—they loved their work, they felt a vocation for medicine that in some ways was "a heart for the work" (Wendland 2010, 177), and they strived to provide health to all. But they also suffered the structural and deliberate abuses of the medical system and were affected by larger forms of violence across the country, which left them feeling powerless. This duality and the strongly competing and opposing centrifugal forces fostered a deep resentment and anger toward the larger system.

I examine the intersection of physicians with public life—specifically as vectors of dissent in two key protests, one in 1964 and another fifty years later in 2014. The broader politics of health, the changing health policies, the legal issues they have faced, and the ways that they have been victims of criminal violence all impact doctors' practice. These structures reproduce in medical spaces, resulting in harsh ways of training such as the use of humiliation, abuse, and punishment by the medical hierarchy. These abuses occurred both in front of patients and behind the scenes in purely medical spaces, blurring the boundary between frontstage and backstage medical performances of the self. All these factors shape clinicians' love (or hate) for what they do and their ability to practice medicine within this harsh context.

FROM SOCIAL SECURITY TO NEOLIBERAL REFORMS

In the book's introduction I briefly discussed the history of medicine in Mexico and how some of the post-revolution ideals were never truly realized in practice. This gap between revolutionary ideals and reality is especially the case for the practice of medicine in public hospitals, where the broader structures are historically reproduced in health systems, creating abusive environments for the workers and reproducing this abuse down the hierarchy to be ultimately enacted on patients. Here I examine this gap, elaborating on some of the ways that broader globalizing forces have shaped the experiences of medical care in Mexico.

The labor of Mexican physicians, as well as their education and practice, have all been shaped over the past 200 years by the country's broader policies. Structurally, Mexico has a complex institutional framework devoted to the health care of its citizens that functions alongside an educational system engaged in the training and education of a professional medical class. Like other Latin American countries, it has a mix of private and public care, and its health-care coverage has historically been based on the social security model, which was meant to reach universal coverage through the economic benefits of modernization (Vargas-Bustamante and Méndez 2014).

Physicians in Mexico have had different relationships with the state (Nigenda and Solórzano 1997), with the first half of the twentieth century consisting of significant autonomy before the establishment of large-scale health institutes, which subordinated their profession to government bureaucracy (Finkler 2004). In the decades immediately surrounding World War II, Mexico experienced a period of unprecedented economic development and prosperity, termed Mexico's "economic miracle"—even though it did not necessarily benefit all people equally (Pensado 2013). During this time there was an emphasis on addressing some of the social justice expectations of the revolution in the form of health and other social support to state workers, union workers, teachers, and others (Soto Laveaga 2015). The country invested an enormous amount of money in the construction of medical infrastructure for the Security and Social Services for Workers of the State (ISSSTE) and Mexican Institute for Social Security (IMSS) hospital systems and in building several very large hospitals to attend to the population. By the mid-twentieth century, the state had primary control of health care and medical education.[3]

This growth in infrastructure was not matched by a growth in the rates of medical student education and graduation (Cabello-López et al. 2015). There were too few health-care workers in hospitals to attend to the increased number of patients. The internship became a stopgap measure to increase the number of health-care providers. Trainees were assigned to take on greater roles in medical care, and they were expected to understand and appreciate hospital medicine. By the end of the century, however, these medical schools had developed an open-door policy for anyone wanting to study medicine, which meant that the country faced the opposite problem: many physicians were produced, leading to a deep class division in the profession. More privileged physicians (usually specialists) maintained an independent foothold in their practice and in their ability to be in leadership positions, while large numbers of doctors (usually general practitioners) were unable to find jobs, resulting in high unemployment and underemployment rates for the profession (see also Finkler 2004). Although doctors were part of the professional class and medicine was seen as a means to expedite the country's social and economic development, this hierarchy between privileged and less-privileged physicians became an important catalyst that channeled a growing dissatisfaction with the medical system.

AWASH IN WHITE: THE 1964–1965 DOCTORS' STRIKE

From the start of the very first cohort of interns in 1962, there were issues between them, the institutions they labored in, and the state, including disagreements about remuneration for their hard labor, their designation as students rather than employees (and the few benefits in the system from being the former), their provision of room and board (Frenk, Hernández-Llamas, and Alvarez-Klein 1983), the different work conditions and pay scales between each hospital type, and the way that many interns were kept in "overworked isolation" (Soto Laveaga 2013a, 32).

The nation's plan of health care for all was achieved through the labor of the less powerful in hospitals—the trainees. Over time interns and residents felt the increased weight of their duties with little recompense or stability. They filled the gaps that attending physicians could not fill. Because they were not salaried employees, they received no benefits or social security, and they had no legal right to complain (Cabello-López et al. 2015). Many felt exploited by the system. This dissatisfaction erupted in 1964 as residents and interns in Mexico City went on strike to protest their working conditions. Their demands emerged from perceptions and values about dignity in the human condition—better salaries, legal contracts, and better working conditions.

Accounts of the strike are quite consistent. It began on November 26, 1964, at one of the newest ISSSTE hospitals in the country.[4] Frustrated trainees formed the Mexican Association of Medical Residents and Interns (AMMRI) and officially presented their demands to the state: an improvement in their labor contracts for better terms and wages, the right to be active participants in the development of their educational curriculum, and a preferential option for being hired as physicians at the institutions of their residency. Additionally, they wanted the state's assurance that they would have the right to return to their posts at the conclusion of the strike without repercussions or reprisals (Cabello Lopez et al. 2015).

Over the course of the next ten months, doctors marched peacefully in the streets of the city, "painting them white" with their uniforms (Archundia-García 2011, S29, my translation). The main organizers were shadowed by agents from the Federal Security Directorate for several months (Soto Laveaga 2013a). In January 1965 the federal government announced that it would begin legal proceedings against interns and residents who had abandoned their posts at emergency hospitals. These threats were followed by a disinformation campaign by the media, controlled by the government, that suggested that the doctors' demands were frivolous and influenced by communism. Rather than these repressions shutting down the protests, they generated increased solidarity. The numbers swelled in protest, including nurses and hospital directors, who supported AMMRI and their strike. Most significantly, this movement, at first localized to Mexico City, spread throughout the country. With mounting public pressure, the country's incoming president Gustavo Díaz Ordaz decreed an end to the strike in early February, seeming to accede to some of the protesters' economic and labor demands. These promises were later broken, prompting even more physicians to join the protests.

In April, the federal government made a public ultimatum, published in newspapers across the country, that if trainees did not return to work by May of that year all negotiations would cease, their jobs would be terminated, and they would be replaced by other personnel (Cabello-López et al. 2015; Gutiérrez-Samperio 2016). Additionally, as historian Gabriela Soto Laveaga (2013a) stated, the government-controlled media portrayed the protesters as unprofessional doctors who were placing the country's welfare at risk. This situation culminated with the protesters doing a silent march to the seat of the federal government in Mexico City.

As Soto Laveaga (2013a) wrote, around this time the protesters began to realize that they were being treated the same way as other groups in the country that sought redress for social justice issues, such as peasant groups, students, and labor unions. For much of the strike the doctors had capitalized on their more privileged status of healers and educated professionals, and so had portrayed their struggle as a just cause. In her research on declassified government documents, Soto Laveaga (2013a) showed how the protesters began to shift to using more radical language, positioning themselves against the state, and connecting their right to strike with the health of the nation (*por la salud del pueblo*).

In June, the leaders of the alliance met again with Díaz Ordaz to reach an end to the strike, but he prevaricated between support for the rights of doctors and distaste for their methods of protest. In response, they organized the largest—and, as it turned out, final—strike (Gutiérrez-Samperio 2016). Protests broke out across the country. About fifty ISSSTE clinics and hospitals across the nation signed letters in support of the strike (Pozas Horcasitas 1993). In Puebla, about 250 students from one of the medical schools and forty-nine residents and physicians from one of the main city hospitals supported their peers in protest.

The Mexican government saw these protests in the same light as protests from university students that had been occurring since the mid-1950s, which were classified as subversive threats to the nation (Pensado 2013, 84), although in reality they were a threat to the hegemony of the ruling party. Reprisals from the government were swift and severe—the entrance of riot police into several large hospitals across the country, the expulsion of key organizers from their posts, blacklisting participants so they could never be hired again, and threats to the protesters and their replacement with military medical personnel (Gutiérrez-Samperio 2016). These government tactics were honed during these protests, which were reprised few years later in even more violent fashion in the brutal massacre of hundreds of students and bystanders on October 2, 1968, in Mexico City.

In his state of the union address, President Díaz Ordaz accused the medical protesters of criminal behavior, including abandonment of their posts, a lack of professional responsibility, incitement to crime, and potentially having caused the deaths of patients due to dereliction of duties. Soto Laveaga (2011) stated that Díaz Ordaz classified the protest as an "act of homicide" because the doctors had failed to live up to their sworn duty to protect the lives of the population. Government reprisals prompted the end of the strike on September 5, 1965, and return to work by most of the protesters. But the end of the strike did not happen without repercussions—about 500 physicians, residents, and interns were fired from their jobs, and sixty had apprehension orders against them (Cabello-Lopez et al. 2015). Tragically, despite the almost year-long strike to change working conditions for the most vulnerable health-care workers, when the interns and residents returned to their hospitals their labor contracts were almost identical to those they had before (Cabello Lopez et al. 2015), causing "a stagnation in the search for equality and justice within the health system" (Casas-Patiño, Reséndiz-Rivera, and Casas 2009, 12, my translation). Despite the obvious outrage felt by the protesters in the 1960s and the lighting of what Archundia-García (2011, S29, my translation) calls a "citizen consciousness" that carried into the 1960s student movements, memories of the medical strike have almost been swallowed by history.

WORKING WITH WHAT WE HAVE

Suspicion between the government and the medical establishment has continued to the present day. In addition, feelings of vulnerability have been exacerbated by drug-related violence throughout Mexico, which has resulted in a pervasive perception of insecurity across the country, affecting all segments of society. For doctors the violence has fueled fears of what it means to practice medicine in twenty-first century Mexico. Over the past few years there have been high-profile kidnappings, disappearances, and brutal murders of doctors and other medical personnel (O'Connor and Booth 2010; Santana 2013) across the country because of internecine violence between drug cartels. Some of this violence has taken place in rural, more remote areas, while others have taken place in the wards of urban hospitals, turning them into war zones (O'Connor and Booth 2010). Many doctors have felt abandoned by the infrastructure that protected them when they were students, and they feel at the mercy of organized crime. In some cases doctors have been kidnapped to provide care to members of the drug cartel (El Economista 2015). Clinics in some regions of the country stand empty, as clinicians refuse to staff them until their safety is guaranteed (Padilla 2018).

Medical care in Mexico is unequally distributed (Finkler 2001; Frenk 2006), and, as one of the directors at Hospital Piedad said, citing Article 4 in the Mexican Constitution, all people have the right to health protection: "Even though the law says they have the right to health, the reality is that not all [Mexicans have access]."

Almost everyone I spoke with unquestionably placed most of the blame for the issues in the medical system squarely on the government. Amanda put it bluntly when she said, "The government steals the money, and there is no budget, and there's nothing for medicine or anything." Diana agreed, saying that the problem was endemic corruption within government; "If the government bothered to provide an adequate infrastructure toward health care in Mexico, I think that we could improve on many, many things." Most people quickly differentiated between the infrastructure in public hospitals and in private ones, because as one female doctor at Piedad said, "Things in private ones are fine, but in the public ones there's nothing."

When my interlocutors spoke about the *sistema médico mexicano* (Mexican health care system) they exclusively meant the public system because private institutions "don't fall within the Mexican system." The stark division between public and private hospitals is evident in both the care for patients and the lives of clinicians within them. Every single participant mentioned the infrastructural issues in public hospitals and the poor patient to doctor ratio. As Aarón said, "It's not the same to attend to six patients in four hours as eighteen patients in four hours." Diana expressed her anger at the inequities within the system:

> Doctors are exploited much more in a public hospital: excessive work shifts [and] seeing many, many patients in a short time period. I feel that many of the doctors in a public hospital are not sufficiently motivated to attend to their patients because they know that they don't earn well, that they don't sleep well, and that they fight with everyone. . . . But not in a private [hospital] . . . because there the timetables and the salaries are well established, [and] the hospital's environment is different. I feel that doctors here [at Hospital Piedad] work more comfortably.

Participants wished the government would allocate more funds to hospitals "so maybe the number of people would reduce as they would not all be amassed in only one [hospital]; the quality [of care] would improve." In Puebla this situation was only exacerbated when one of the city's largest public hospitals was severely damaged by a powerful earthquake on September 19, 2017, which destroyed and damaged thousands of buildings across central Mexico. This hospital had 415 beds and attended to over 60 percent of Puebla's IMSS-eligible population (Aroche 2019). Its patients had to be attended at other IMSS hospitals, severely straining the existing resources, with one report concluding that some services were at 300 percent capacity (Castillo 2018).[5]

Severely strained resources occurred in most public hospitals, some of which had equipment that did not work, so patients would have to be sent to other hospitals. Kevin from Hospital Salud said that in his experience some public hospitals were fine and had the necessary equipment for medical personnel to carry out their duties, but that others were more "unkempt in terms of cleanliness, their physical appearance, the installations, and the services." Doctor García, an obstetrician at Hospital Piedad, said that he never wanted to work in a public hospital because of the infrastructural issues but also because "I never liked the treatment towards patients. . . . Unfortunately, the Mexican medical system is overflowing and the doctors are very tired, in a bad mood, and that makes them treat their patients badly." Patients often blame physicians for these situations, and, as Julieta, from Hospital Piedad, said, "What they don't know is that there are twenty people after them also waiting for treatment." Most interlocutors said that the country needed to invest in more physicians in public hospitals so they would have the time to care for them "because you can't reduce the number of patients."

One recurring complaint among my interlocutors was that in some public clinics and hospitals there was a marked lack of supplies (Finkler 2001). One intern said that public hospitals "have nothing. . . . They don't have gloves, there are no face masks, no catheters; that's the problem: a lack of supplies." Amanda mentioned that one of her external rotations was at an IMSS clinic that was so underfunded that they lacked basic supplies such as cotton swabs, alcohol, needles, and gloves. She said that they had to use the same scalpel for every patient, only cleaning it with hydrogen peroxide between patients: "If I'm only given one scalpel a week, what do I do? It's not as though I can tell the patient, 'come back next week.'" She added that this practice shocked her because in medical school they had been taught "that there are some things that you use for one patient only, like a scalpel, a needle, and those things that you can get really sick from [a] patient." She added, "I think it's terrible even if it's free," and that maybe patients needed to be told to bring the missing supplies when they came for care. Another intern added that she felt that it was up to the politicians to provide effective budgets to public hospitals so they could have many supplies because in those institutions "they count your gloves. You have ten patients, and you have to do ten procedures. You have eight pairs of gloves." When I asked what she did under those circumstances, she said she would have to spend her own money to buy gloves. As another intern concluded, people "improvise as best they can."

Scarcity of supplies was only one part (see Ureste 2016b). My interlocutors spoke about a scarcity of medications, physicians, and specialists. Sebastián stated, "There are hospitals but they don't have physicians nor supplies. [Hospitals] are just decorative." Diana said, "So we have to depend on or resign ourselves to what we have, and many times you can make a good diagnostic with a good physical examination. . . . And you know there are many things that could be improved, but that you know would be very hard to do." Doctor Marco, a first-year resident at Hospital Salud, put it most succinctly when he said, "here we work with what we have, not with what we would like to have."

The vicious cycle of care in public hospitals was firmly tied to the high number of patients. The more patients there were, the harder it was for physicians to care for them, and the greater likelihood they would mistreat them. Although in any institution there are rogue providers, the bulk of the practitioners I met wanted to provide good care to their patients; the health-care structure prevented them from doing so. A consequence of the high number of patients was that the wait times were very long, sometimes extending for months "for everything: consults, procedures, lab work, surgeries," including tests and treatment for patients suffering from cancer or other acute conditions. These "clinical temporalities" (Andaya 2019, 652) were encapsulated in a joke told by some of my participants: "Imagine if abortion becomes legal in Mexico. You go to the [public hospital] to get an appointment, and by the time it's your turn the little blessing is in first grade."

Elise Andaya (2019) suggested that the ways that time is managed in clinics reproduces racism/status difference within these institutions, whereby some populations wait while others do not. Building on Javier Auyero's (2012) work on the different ways that the Argentine state makes impoverished populations wait, Andaya concluded that the poor are expected to wait because they should be grateful for the charity care they receive (657). As my interlocutors reminded me, "In private hospitals there is no wait time. Everything is instantaneous." Doctors working in private care "spoil their patients" because they pay for care and "[as a doctor] you limit yourself to what the patient wants." Kevin described private care as having luxurious service, equipment, and available procedures. He also said that the care was better because "they have to be more attentive, they have to be more obliging. I say 'have to' because [doctors] are obliged to do that because you are paying for a service and good care."

If, as they stated, private hospitals are "outside" of the Mexican health-care system, there is an additional stratification of care that impacts the most needy. In such a situation those who are economically privileged can afford to be apart from the rest of Mexico, and, as Rosalynn Vega (2018, 189) suggested, they can position themselves as consumers within transnational networks, an option that "is just out of reach" to the bulk of the population dependent on public care. As Diana concluded, "Public care should be the same as private [care] even if the patient is not paying for it. Because, after all, it's medicine. Medicine should not be different whether it's public or private, because after all, it's not as though you have public and private appendicitis, right?" Laughing ruefully, she added, "It should be the same, equitable, and it's definitely not like that. And it's so many things that would be really very hard work to change."

THE VIOLENCE OF HUMILIATION: TOXIC HIERARCHIES

The violence of this system was reproduced between the clinicians in the medical spaces, particularly within the medical hierarchy, resulting in toxic hierarchies that greatly affected people's ability to practice good medicine. Medicine has what Johan Galtung (1990) calls a steep Self–Other gradient; that is, because the hierarchy is so marked, those at the top are powerful, and those at the bottom are othered and stripped of power. The hierarchy of medical and social relations means that people's self-identity changes depending on the social context (Scheper-Hughes and Lock 1987). Although hierarchies are not inherently problematic, when a hierarchy is exploited by those at the top, it tends to reproduce violent structures. People's "inner processes are shaped amid violence, political domination, and social suffering" (Biehl, Good, and Kleinman 2007, 1).

As Castro and Villanueva Lozano (2018) have stated, most doctors are very aware of the external violence that affects them—policy changes, lawsuits, or violence against the self from criminals. They argue that doctors are often hypersensitive to behaviors and perceived violence that undermine their medical respectability and practice, including things that are not usually considered to be violent (like a lawsuit). They add that doctors frequently conflate legitimate actions of the state, as reflected by policies and ministerial actions, with the illegitimate acts of criminals (such as kidnapping or murder of medical personnel), and respond to both of these different forms of violence as equal assaults on their profession. In their study, Castro and Villanueva Lozano (2018) concluded that doctors are much less aware of the systemic and symbolic violence internal to medical spaces, and they unthinkingly enact or incorporate this violence into their practice. Symbolic violence is usually manifested in contexts of power differentials, where both the powerful and the powerless groups unconsciously participate in enacting the norms imposed by those with greater power (Bourdieu and Wacquant 1992); these assumptions underlie people's beliefs and practices.

The incongruence of doctors being hypervigilant of external violence while failing to recognize or acknowledge internal violence occurs commonly in medicine, where doctors frequently have coexisting but contrasting systems that they have to resolve in practice (Castro and Villanueva Lozano 2018), such as the tussle between caring for patients but not becoming emotionally involved, or having to learn hands-on practice with patients but spending most of their time on paperwork away from patients. As doctors learn that medical training can be aggressive and brutal, they also learn to not question the violence and to classify violent behaviors as normal. Violence recedes into the background of the formal curriculum and communicates to the trainees what is actually valued in medicine.

Although not all doctors are abusive or have been abused, the trend is toward an abusive system. Symbolic violence is present in interactions as well as in how language is deployed (Žižek 2008) to reinforce the domination of one group and the subordination of another, bringing about potentially serious harms to subordinates. This abuse happens at all levels. Those lower on the hierarchy are told or made to feel that "they are lower" or "they barely matter." Galtung (1990) proposed the concept of "cultural violence" to articulate those aspects of a culture that are deployed to legitimate or justify violence; he argued that this form of violence makes direct and structural violence feel and look right.

Those at the bottom of the hierarchy are most aware of the violence and give voice to their concerns. Regina from Hospital Piedad said that when she first entered the internship the ranks were very marked and the more senior interns were empowered by one of the directors to be more assertive—and this translated into abuse. We had a very emotional conversation where she spoke about how much she loved medicine and how she felt it was her vocation, but that she had struggled considerably with interpersonal dynamics and bullying during the internship. Tears running down her cheek, she said that the senior interns considered themselves to be superior and would tell her "you go and do this and this and this." She added that she found surgery to be one of the hardest rotations: "So, I remember that . . . they would give me a ton of things [to do] and I could see them resting in the residence doing nothing or watching movies. And if I was missing something [they would say], 'You didn't finish this; how can you be so irresponsible!'" Other interns in her cohort agreed. Julieta said that this abuse was transmitted down the hierarchy: "The attending to the resident; and the resident to the intern; and the intern to the *internito* (junior intern). . . . In all this environment it's like that. The hierarchies are very, very, very marked." She added that her cohort made a concerted effort not to be abusive to their juniors because it was not productive for anyone. She sighed and said that her aim was to change the system as "it should be a friendlier environment between us . . . including nurses, interns, residents, doctors."

Doctor Juan, a kind and gentle resident at Hospital Piedad, spoke at length about the hierarchical nature of the medical system and the toxicity that this created. As he spoke, he sat back comfortably in his chair, playing distractedly with a staple on the table. He emphasized the presence of humiliation and mistreatment and how, as one moved up the hierarchy, the humiliation to those below intensified to the point that the highest ranked residents were godlike, where junior residents "don't even have the right to look at them." He believed this culture affected people's performance and labor. He stated that this was a long-standing generational form of teaching "where you have to treat and pressure your resident below you or even the intern so they study more, read more. . . . It's almost like a militarized system, right? I do think it's good to demand [hard work] or for [someone] to demand [hard work] from you. That is excellent. But the form it takes needs to change."

He described one instance when the residents had strongly scolded the interns for not knowing about a certain class of medications: "I mean, if you tell them, 'you made a mistake in this, this, and this; start studying' but you say it in a good way, nothing happens. On the contrary, you motivate them to work hard and to improve. But if you scold them and you mistreat them, they get frustrated, and what they want is to drop out of school or leave the internship. . . . Many physicians abandon the residency because of the pressure, because of all they have to study, the work they have to do, and they desert it because of the pressure." In this narrative Doctor Juan distinguished between harsh forms of instruction and the combination of hierarchy and abuse. The latter becomes a much greater issue with trainees because it can have enormous repercussions on people's physical and mental well-being—as has been the case with several trainees in Mexico who have committed suicide (Olvera 2019). Additionally, Doctor Juan emphasized that an important aspect to any structure and hierarchy was respect, but that when respect was demanded of those lower on the hierarchy (and was not accorded to them in turn), this was a problem. He considered this a human rights issue whereby "in the hospital [and] outside of it, our rights are the same."

Although the country has prohibited hazing and punishments of medical trainees, the behaviors continue. In 2013 the State of Puebla's Commission for Human Rights (Comisión de Derechos Humanos del Estado de Puebla [CDHP] 2015) launched an investigation into these issues and concluded that there was evidence that 81 percent of trainees had experienced cruel, heartless, or degrading treatment, sometimes in front of patients or other hospital colleagues, 69 percent had experienced physical or psychological violence, and 67 percent felt that their rights had been violated. Many of them had been punished with extra-long shifts. Additional abuses identified in other studies included refusing to teach "problematic" trainees, preventing trainees from eating or using the bathroom, pressuring trainees to consume alcohol against their will, and using physical violence on trainees. Unsurprisingly, trainees experienced burnout, depression, anxiety, or suicidal ideation/actions, and they also sometimes took out their frustration on their patients through poor care (Derive et al. 2018; Montes-Villaseñor et al. 2018). These were accepted forms of culturally violent behavior in many medical spaces; although trainees might have grumbled to each other about the violence, they also perceived it as a natural part of training, inherent to their formation as medical professionals.

DOLING OUT CASTIGOS

One morning in the obstetrics ward at Hospital Salud I could hear the residents and interns laughing loudly in the *Cuarto de Médicos,* the Doctor's Room. It was a small, windowless, stuffy space outfitted with one twin bed with a rumpled set of sheets, which served as both bed and sofa, two scuffed desks, two old desktop computers, a printer, a small fridge, and a wall clock that did not work. Residents' and interns' backpacks crammed with their street clothes littered the floor or were piled haphazardly on a bench. White coats hung droopily on a rack above the bed. On hot days the air barely moved in the ward and seemed to willfully stagnate in the Cuarto. When I peeked in, I saw Nicolás, a short, stocky intern, doing a funny chicken-like dance and wiggling his bottom. Everyone was laughing hysterically.

I had never seen them so relaxed. Doctor Marco, a junior resident, and Doctora Valentina, a senior resident, were seated by the computer; she would occasionally scroll through YouTube for music, but did not play anything for long. Doctora Valentina was one of the hardest working residents in the ward. With the interns she had a good joking relationship, though she would rapidly become stern if she was displeased. With her male peers she had cultivated a playful relationship, responding to their punching or teasing in kind. Doctor Bruno, another junior resident, lay on the bed charging his phone with Doctor Marco's cord, and he distractedly pulled at the lace of a disposable boot peeking out of a locker. Nicolás sat down next to him and soon fell fast asleep. Bianca, a petite intern with long black hair and large glasses in dark frames, sat on the bench and motioned for Megan and me to join her.

Thus far in our interactions I had been the one to ask them questions about medical training in Mexico; on this day they turned the tables and began to inquire about medical school in the United States. They were amazed at some of the structures (the shorter hours, the low patient to doctor ratio, the large beds) and were aghast at others (especially the tuition). We soon began to talk about their long shifts, and they said that residents usually arrived at the hospital by 7:00 A.M. and left by 6:00 P.M. (the interns left at 3:00 P.M.). In other specialties the residents were expected to stay until all the work was done. As they spoke, I noticed Doctor Bruno and Doctor Marco using the respect form of "*usted*" rather than the informal "*tú*" when speaking to Doctora Valentina, who was their senior. This was common practice for interns toward residents, nurses, and attending doctors; although it reflected the respectful ways of common speech in Mexico, it also reflected the symbolic violence of how language was deployed in these spaces, where most residents were all approximately the same age and it was only rank that differentiated how they spoke and interacted with each other. Among the interns I met, Bianca seemed to be the only one who broke protocol, using "*tú*" for Doctor Marco, who seemed to invite more informality.[6]

After a while, Doctor Bruno asked Doctora Valentina whether he could leave the ward to have a meal; with her permission he left. Doctor Marco joked that they had the next thirty-six hours to spend together. Bianca expressed nervousness about one of the senior doctors because "he scares me." When Doctor Marco asked why, she said that he scolded and shouted a lot, and when she did something wrong he would yell out for the nurse to come in to replace her. Doctor Marco pragmatically told her, "One learns something from all of them." He added that the same doctor had also shouted at him about his skills with the instruments or about not doing some things correctly. Doctora Valentina joined the conversation and they began to talk about *castigos*—the punishments notorious in many public hospitals across the country.

I had heard about some of these castigos in my conversations with participants, such as indirect punishments for "lazy" trainees who would be assigned the additional physical labor of fetching and carrying materials, paperwork, or patients; or trainees who had made mistakes and would be asked to bring in pizza, sushi, or "*pollo Kentucky*" for the team; or, the mildest form, most closely aligned with actual medical learning, where trainees were required to study a topic that they had not known when questioned by a senior clinician. Kevin, one of the other interns at Hospital Salud, had earlier described the system to me as "old school," wherein interns were sometimes taught to learn through fear by being scolded, and "*a los golpes*," which literally translates as "by brute/physical force." The latter here likely refers to aggressive or forcible teaching such as the mano dura I explored in chapter 1, as illustrated by César telling his peers that he had received a "*madreada*" (slang meaning to beat someone up, but here describing a severe reprimand) by one of the attending doctors because Julieta had not filled out a form correctly. However, learning "a los golpes" was also present as a form of literal physical violence, such as when residents like Doctor Enrique from Hospital Salud were known to use clamps to hit trainees when they made mistakes, as I described in the last chapter. These practices, along with psychological and symbolic violence, were seen to be a means to "form people's characters." Kevin described how residents considered castigos as something that "should [either] hurt you or cost you." During another conversation years later, when he was about to start his residency at an IMSS hospital, he joked about a meme that said "Many congratulations to everyone chosen to begin their residency this year; be happy and don't worry, the R1 [first year] is a party. And you are the piñata."

On this day, the residents and interns began to describe some of the harsher castigos present in their training and in other hospitals. I heard about trainees who had been given "guardias de castigo" and forced to stay additional hours (or days) in the hospital as punishment for mistakes or transgressions, and new residents who had been expected to stay for two weeks straight "to get used to the hospital." I also later heard about another case, described in several news sources, about a surgical resident at a different Puebla hospital who experienced a strong example of mano dura training: he was given the option of being sequestered at the hospital for two months or putting on boxing gloves and fighting another resident; he chose the latter and sustained a hematoma that required surgery (Olvera 2019). Doctora Valentina said that when she was a first-year resident at Hospital Salud the senior residents prohibited her from using the elevator. She laughed and said she did not mind using the stairs: "anyway, it's only one floor up." She did worry about the guardias and felt that residents were abused because they spent so much time in the hospital. She felt that "it's not that good for the patients for us to be so tired."

Their lighthearted mood prevailed, however, and they soon began to laugh about a senior resident who was known to be brutal in his treatment of everyone subordinate to him and of doling out punishments regularly. They described how one time he was very upset at some of the junior residents (including Doctor Bruno) and punished them by not allowing them into a surgery. They said that he took two interns instead, but did not let them do anything. They laughed about how he almost did the surgery with his feet as he performed everything himself. Medical bioethicist Katie Watson (2011) stated that being off balance can make one laugh "and sometimes laughing is what keeps us from falling over." Their seemingly lighthearted laughter served to hide or diminish the darker symbolic violence that this doctor enacted on the most vulnerable—like being the piñata for those of higher ranks. It exposed the hegemony in the violence, maintaining and not questioning the hierarchical order of the hospital.

Because the medical system is a meritocracy, it bestows authority on those at the top, who can then wield power over the "more unworthy" or "less meritorious" people below. The abuses that my interlocutors experienced, and those uncovered by other scholars and news sources, often occur frontstage rather than backstage (Goffman 1959), in both public and private spaces, in front of patients and in front of other clinicians. They blurred the boundary between front and backstage actions and performances, although rarely did they seem to take place offstage, behind closed doors. Humiliations and castigos were a performance of medical authority from those in power to those who were only just cultivating a medical self, and they *had* to take place before an audience. The senior resident who had banished the residents performed the role of a godlike doctor who could single-handedly (or footedly, to use the humor of the residents) manage a complex surgery. The doctors who had forced the residents at other hospitals to don boxing gloves or endure guardias de castigo were performing their authority to control not only the individual bodies of the junior residents but also the broader social body of the medical wards. By imposing these punishments, doctors were able to remind and demonstrate to others how they were meant to behave, and to reinforce that they were expected to follow the rules and expectations of this space.

Doctors in training and those above them embody two identities within these spaces. On the one hand, they are agents within the hospital, able to exert power (if they want) over those lower on the hierarchy and over patients; they experience upward mobility, with each rung in the hierarchy shedding part of their vulnerability in their journey toward medical expertise. On the other hand, they are powerless in the face of abuses in the system. This duality between the ordinary and extraordinary present within medicine creates friction that continues to define and give shape to trainees' medical selves. In the process they learn how to balance these competing narratives and forces. Many of them learn to acquire and foster a medical self that enables them to wield knowledge as power, to move up the system and become experts.

NEITHER GODS NOR CRIMINALS:
THE 2014 MEDICAL PROTESTS

The 2014 medical protests had both structural and immediate causes. Their substrate was the ongoing and problematic labor conditions of hospital staff across the country and the planned implementation of a new universal health care system that was to have cost and service sharing between the major health systems (IMSS, ISSSTE, and Ministry of Health). Patients would be able to go to any public hospital and receive free care; all they needed was their national identification. Physicians such as Doctor Jesús Morales, a portly doctor from Hospital Piedad who always wore a suit under his white coat, were concerned that this new system would amplify the current limits to health care that Mexico faced because it would stretch resources to their breaking point. He deeply cared about making sure interns were becoming professionals. As Gabriel, a very hard working and competent intern at Hospital Piedad, said, many doctors were in support of care for all, but the government seemed to forget that Mexico was not a wealthy European country.

The additional substrate was that the continued drug-related violence affected doctors, especially as the state mandated that all medical students perform a year of social service in underserved regions, some of which were known to be dangerous and where doctors had already been victims of violence. For instance, in 2010 clinicians from seventeen hospitals and clinics in Ciudad Juárez, across the U.S.–Mexico border from El Paso, Texas, suspended their labor for twenty-four hours in protest of the violence their *compañeros* had suffered; in that year alone, eleven medical personnel had been kidnapped, two of whom were murdered, and countless other clinicians were subject to extortion (Villalpando and Breach 2010). As part of their protest, clinicians organized die-ins where participants wore blood-spattered white coats and held signs with the names of the victims.

The immediate causes of the 2014 protests were sparked by an arrest order in 2014 issued by a judge against sixteen physicians in an IMSS hospital in the state of Jalisco for the death of a fifteen-year-old patient in 2010.[7] Two sides to this conflict emerged. One side consisted of the patient's family and much of the mainstream media, which alleged that the boy had entered the hospital in late 2009 with what seemed to be an asthmatic crisis, possibly caused by the H1N1 flu virus. After some tests, the diagnosis was discarded, although the tests might have caused the perforation of both lungs. Attention then shifted to the patient's intestines, as doctors believed he had a perforation. Over the next two weeks the young patient underwent more than half a dozen surgical interventions, including resections, which according to some media sources were not sent to a pathologist (Rello 2014). He lost approximately four liters of blood and never regained consciousness. Fifty-five days after admittance to the hospital, he died. An autopsy by a forensic medical team revealed that he had died from intestinal tuberculosis rather than the intestinal sepsis listed as the cause on the IMSS-issued death certificate.[8]

Physicians and the IMSS workers' union, on the other hand, saw this situation as an effort to criminalize medical practitioners and as a way for the patient's family to make money from the lawsuit. The executive committee for the IMSS workers' union defended the physicians, stating that by the time the patient was taken to the hospital after having been seen by other medical systems, he was cyanotic and in respiratory and cardiac arrest, needing to be revived through CPR. He was moved into the ICU where several different specialists examined him, concluding that he had an intestinal perforation, which was addressed by surgery. The report from the syndicate ends abruptly, omitting several of the details given by the other sources, including the fact that the patient spent almost two months in the hospital. It states, "Despite the multiple medical and surgical treatments carried out by the medical specialists, the patient's extremely critical status continued deteriorating until it concluded in the unfortunate death several days after his hospital admission" (Radio Formula 2017).

The truth about the boy's death and about the role the doctors played was likely somewhere between these extremes, which pitted doctors and patients against each other (see Soto Laveaga and Agostoni 2011). After the 2014 arrest warrants were issued, doctors at the Jalisco IMSS launched a Twitter campaign to support their colleagues with the hashtag #YoSoy17 (I am 17).[9] They denounced the aggressions toward doctors, both the legal and drug-related violence, demanded that medical actions should not be criminalized or legally sanctioned, and appealed to the state to guarantee their safety when performing their duties. The idea behind the campaign was that any doctor could be the seventeenth member of the accused group because they had all been in a similar position at some time or another. What began as a simple call to support their colleagues went viral, growing into a nationwide protest about problematic hospital labor conditions.

Doctors defended their practices and claimed that patient deaths and accusations of iatrogenesis were not their fault but were caused by unfair labor conditions—much like their predecessors' strike fifty years earlier.[10] Like the doctors' clinical narratives this chapter began with, these doctors positioned their ordinary medical practice against a backdrop of extraordinary difficulty, where they were victims of the story rather than the agentive protagonists. One article cited a doctor who said, "These are not mistakes; they are from the excessive workloads we have. . . . Everyone knows that it's the excessive workload because the physician is always given that responsibility" (Velazco 2014). People posting on the social media platforms Twitter and Facebook claimed that they were not at fault for patient outcomes because it was a system built against them, with long guardias, limited resources, a high patient load, and corrupt politicians siphoning off funds. Posts on social media included a multitude of slogans. "We're Doctors, Not Gods, Nor Criminals." "We owe ourselves to our patients;

we're physicians thanks to them and for them!!" "Let's dignify our profession without forgetting our commitments to our patients." "For a more humane form of health care for our patients." "Come on indignant and victimized doctors, say your piece." "Errare humanum est [To err is human]." As these slogans indicate, many of the participants in these protests perceived the external violence from the legal system as one that undermined both their role as physicians and the respectability of their profession. Other slogans noted by Castro and Villanueva Lozano (2018), such as "No more violence against health care workers" and "No to the accusation of obstetric violence," illustrate the ways that the protesters conflated different issues as equal forms of external violence.

These online protests eventually materialized in real life when doctors marched in protest on June 22, 2014, in dozens of cities across the nation. As their colleagues had in 1964, these protesters wore their white coats and carried signs, but they added a black ribbon around their upper arm to mark the violence experienced by members of their profession. Videos taken of these marches show city avenues awash with white coats (Aristegui Noticias 2014). One national newspaper headline referred to the #YoSoy17 campaign as "The death of a young man that unleashed a national movement" (Excélsior 2014, my translation).

WE NEED TO CHANGE THE WHOLE SYSTEM

The doctors' marches have been repeated since 2014 on a yearly basis or even more frequently, and they have sometimes also occurred in pockets across the nation on October 23, National Doctors' Day in Mexico. These protests have brought to the surface a long-standing tussle between policy-makers and practitioners, patients and doctors. Researchers have shown that the funds provided to the health-care and education sectors are insufficient to combat both long-standing diseases and emerging ones. Significant cutting of expenses considered superfluous—including medical training and research—has been prevalent and has only increased since the devastating 1985 earthquake in Mexico City destroyed several hospitals (García Procel 2007).

While government funds for health care have been reduced yearly, making it harder for practitioners to do their work, there has been a simultaneous concern from policy-makers and government ministries with the quality of care provided to patients. As one of the leaders of the protest stated in a speech, "We ask [the Minister of Health] to actually see the shortage of supplies, the scarcity, the lack of upkeep and maintenance of the [medical] units; we ask them to recognize the work conditions that forced our colleagues in Jalisco to fall into that situation" (Enciso 2014, my translation). The speaker added that recurring punitive action against "the medical class" forces doctors to work under threat and to remain silent about a problematic medical system. As one of my participants stated, "[I wish doctors] would not make distinctions between patients. That they don't say 'if they pay me more, I'll treat them better, and if they pay me less, I ignore them.' So, yes, to treat everyone the same, because they're all human beings, they all need medical [care]."

In 2016, some of the organizers of the marches presented additional demands to the Minister of Health, which included improved labor conditions, increases in the budget for basic materials such as gauze and sutures, upgrades to the infrastructure of public hospitals, improvements in the safety of medical personnel (Ureste 2016a), and a guarantee of health as a human right for all (Castilllo Yáñez 2016). These ongoing protests can be seen as a friction between the medical and legal systems, where practitioners are feeling increasingly squeezed from all sides. As Soto Laveaga (2013a, 31) stated, the 1960s strike lasted ten months, "but the illusion of contentment among the upwardly mobile classes had been irrevocably broken." The same can be said of the twenty-first century protests. These were protests of a professional class that felt excluded from and abused by the ideals of the revolution and taken advantage of by a system run by extraordinary corruption and violence.

Doctors labored in health institutions originally created for social justice, but they were entirely left out of these ideals (Cabello-López et al. 2015). As most of my participants stated, "We need to reestablish the entire Mexican medical system." In 2019, Mexico's new left-leaning president Andrés Manuel López Obrador (known by his initials of AMLO) did just that. He made sweeping changes to the health system, canceling several long-standing programs, such as the conditional cash transfer program Prospera (originally known as Oportunidades; Smith-Oka 2013b) and Seguro Popular, claiming that the latter was neither secure nor popular ("*que ni es seguro, ni es popular*"). He instead created the National Health Plan, which included the establishment of the National Health Institute for Well-being (INSABI), and he committed to providing almost $2 billion for hospital infrastructure, making health care free and universal, guaranteeing medical supplies, increasing the number of health-care workers, and incentivizing them to work in remote and underserved regions. This very idealized plan struggled from the start, straining the medical system, causing a reduction in supplies and medications, and affecting patients.[11] Small but vocal protests by both health-care workers and patients occurred at several hospitals throughout 2019 and early 2020 in response to these changes and difficulties.

This strained system would be problematic under ordinary circumstances but became catastrophic when hit by COVID-19, the novel coronavirus pandemic, in March 2020. Supplies became increasingly scarce, hospitals' bed capacities reached their limit, and doctors were stressed and overworked (Sherman 2020; Kitroeff and Villegas 2020). Small protests occurred in response to months of difficulties of caring for patients suffering from COVID-19. Larger, nationwide protests were called by mid-2020 in response to violence against doctors—a male emergency doctor in Chiapas was arrested after his politician patient died of the disease, a female doctor in Guerrero was assassinated by unknown assailants, and countless others were harassed and verbally abused. The medical protestors stated that in addition to the lack of medications and too much work, "we feel betrayed when we are not protected" and that "we demand that the authorities apply preventative measures and protect the life of health-care workers, doctors, and nurses, because we are who are responsible for caring for the health and life of the population" (Briseño 2020, my translation). For many of them, the government's response was emblematic of the nation's issues—medicine was a contested space between policy and practice that revived revolutionary promises while simultaneously breaking them on the backs of doctors and patients.

What do trainees learn about being doctors from these situations? How do ordinary and extraordinary parts of medical lives become embodied in their practice? As trainees develop a medical self, they learn to pay active attention to certain things that matter personally to them, while also ignoring those that they do not consider important. Some trainees might create a stronger focus toward the extraordinary and the external—the violence and difficulties affecting their medical self. Others might ignore the external and instead focus on the ordinary self-making practices of medicine—enskilment, competence, or caring. Most, however, find a balance between these extremes, paying attention to some of the external and some of the internal, positioning themselves as competent and caring physicians who are also aware of the broader structural forces shaping medical practice.

3 · THE SOUL OF
THE HOSPITAL
Life as an Intern

We tend to observe the patient in [units], like, "I'm an ophthalmologist, I only see eyes," "I'm an endocrinologist, only hormones," "I'm a surgeon, only [surgery]." I sometimes think that what's needed is to see the whole, complete process.... We should see the patient as integrated.

—Regina, intern at Hospital Piedad

If the doctor sees that you are really useless, he's not going to let you do anything; he might even ask you to leave. But if he sees that you are skilled and you have initiative, he'll probably let you put in the sutures.

—Iker, intern at Hospital Salud

The first-year residents do everything. The ones higher up the hierarchy do nothing; they say they've already done that.... They just devote themselves to scolding.

—Kevin, intern at Hospital Salud

Doctor Antonio Contreras was an elderly, gregarious physician at Hospital Piedad. Beloved by the interns, he was frequently sought out for professional and personal advice, which he relished sharing. Interns would often ask doctors to teach a class on a specific topic; Doctor Contreras's classes were usually an hour-long stream of consciousness about medicine, interspersed with his thoughts on topics ranging from former patients and where one could find the best tacos in Puebla, to his concerns with societal problems, all interspersed with off-color jokes. His medical practice was deeply shaped by his Catholic faith, and he believed that doctors should serve the poor and those less fortunate. He believed in being both a professor and a teacher. Professors, in his view, were those who taught a medical topic, while teachers were those who taught about life and "who reflect with their own life . . . a way of being a doctor." He said that medical students were taught skills but not values: "They'll tell you, 'For *Staphylococcus* prescribe dicloxacillin.' But no one will tell you, 'Don't steal, . . . don't do [expensive tests] for everyone. . . . Don't charge in excess; if you see a person who comes to you barefooted or wearing *huaraches* [woven leather sandals], lower your rates!'" He would make trainees "reflect that the life of the physician is very humanistic; it's not to make money—that comes later—it's not to get power—that also comes later." When he heard what I was researching, he took me under his wing, offering his opinions on medical training, teaching, and hospital life. He described interns to me one day as the "soul of the hospital."

I was drawn to his perception of interns as the animating force of the hospital. During my time shadowing the interns, I saw their formidable labor, where they were up at all hours doing the needful work of the institution. The Greek philosopher Plato considered the relationship between the soul and the body as one of attunement—that the harmony between body and soul is like tuning an instrument (Lan 1995). If interns are the soul of a hospital's body, their labor can then be one of ensoulment, which, while ever present, invisibly exists within the structures of the institution. Paradoxically, when the interns and the hospital are in harmony, the interns' labor remains invisible. When interns are sick or unable to work, their contributions to the institution, by their very absence, become more valued.

In early February 2016, the Popocatepetl, one of the volcanoes that surround Puebla, ejected an enormous plume of ash, which rained down on the city, dusting everything with a thin, snow-like layer. This ash exacerbated a minor flu epidemic in the city, and hospitals were soon overflowing with patients suffering from respiratory ailments. Interns were cautioned to protect themselves with additional hygiene measures as well as mandatory facemasks. One intern personalized his N95 facemask by drawing a dog muzzle on it, making everyone he met smile. On the morning of the eruption, Gabriel from Hospital Piedad texted me, "We're in contingency [mode]," as more than half the interns were sick. Several of the sick interns were at home, and one was hospitalized due to the severity of her illness. As I walked along Piedad's corridors to the emergency ward, I noticed many people coughing. The emergency interns would be moved to other areas of the hospital to cover empty shifts. "I'm worried about the *guardias* [overnight shifts]. Guardia B is empty," said Victoria. Her worry at this sacrifice came both from taking on additional work and from having to practice in unfamiliar areas and skill sets. Knowledge that she would get little sleep added to her dismay.

Hospital training can range from high intensity, where trainees were "on" for hours or even days at a time with little to no rest, to much lower intensity when they studied techniques they hoped to perfect, relaxed with their fellow trainees and shared stories, food, and laughter, or passed out from exhaustion. The life of medical trainees was sometimes ordinary, monotonous, and repetitive— carrying out medical examinations, writing patient medical histories, and taking samples for laboratory tests. This ritualized repetition reinforces the knowledge and practice they are meant to acquire, and it communicates what things are valued in medicine, thereby contributing to a medical self. Michael Jackson (1983) proposed that embodied learning is a practical mimesis "based upon a bodily awareness of the other in oneself" (336). Trainees discover cultural knowledge by themselves as they "fine tune" their perception through observation and mimicry in the process entering into an empathic relationship with a skilled practitioner (Gieser 2008). They gradually learn what the expert knows, maybe even surpassing that person.

This chapter illustrates the tense and productive frictions that inhere in contemporary processes of clinical training, ultimately revealing how interns come to form their medical selves. I focus on the culture within the medical spaces and interactions, particularly how trainees gain enskilment with medical artifacts, how they are taught to approach practice and incorporate values into it, how they are taught to think about patients and case narratives, how mistakes become part of the process of learning, and how all of these are threaded with invisible assumptions about what is good medicine and what makes a good physician. I argue that as trainees form their medical self and acquire expertise, what was once extraordinary gradually shifts to being ordinary.

BECOMING A DOCTOR IN MEXICO

Hospitals as sites for medical training, innovation, and practice are also crucial locations for the production of medical and scientific knowledge (Soto Laveaga 2015). Interns have been incorporated into Mexican hospitals' hallways since 1962, allowing thousands of trainees to face real medical situations (figure 8). All hospitals have *Jefes de Enseñanza* (chiefs of clinical training) responsible for the training of its medical students, interns, and residents. As I described in the book's introduction, medical school in Mexico is six years long, consisting of four years on the university campus followed by a year-long hospital internship.[1] All the interns at Piedad had attended a private medical school in Puebla, while all but one intern at Salud had attended public medical school.[2] The interns I met at both hospitals shared their different pathways to enter medicine (table 1). Some, like Nicolás, had parents who were doctors; some, like Julieta or Iker, saw how doctors had seemed to perform miracles in treating their family members' health; others, like Ricardo, entered medicine because they met doctors who became good role models and who encouraged them to think of medicine as a career; and yet others, like Regina or Kevin, entered medicine because they felt a deep vocation to help people and were committed to questions of social justice.

Though most of the physicians I met loved teaching about medicine, they sometimes expressed disillusionment with the younger generations. Doctor Jesús Morales, a physician in Piedad's emergency room (ER), believed that too many people were allowed into medical school and wished there were stricter

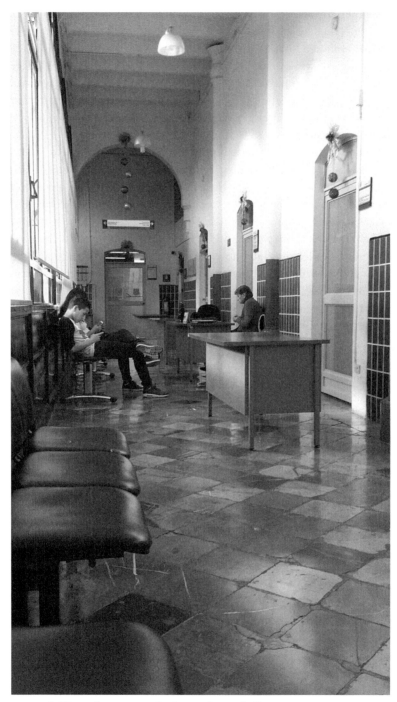

FIGURE 8. Hospital passageway leading to doctors' offices

TABLE 1 Paths to Medicine

Reason for Medical School	Exemplar Quotes	Percentage
Intellectual reasons	"I am really interested in physiology, the why of things, what has to happen for a muscle to contract, to move." (Emilio) In school I always liked . . . natural sciences, biology, chemistry." (Paola) "Primarily the drive to improve myself." (Omar)	29%
Impact of family health issues	"I saw how the doctors helped [my mother]." (César) "[When my grandmother fell sick] I began to realize that one needs a doctor in the family." (Victoria) "My mom had a vascular situation and paralysis on half her body." (Iker)	17%
Family with physicians	"I've had a lot of contract with the profession because both my parents are doctors." (Nicolás)	17%
Vocation	"I began discovering that personal vocation. . . . By combining a social and a religious vocation is my way of reaching God, providing for others." (Regina) "I decided to study medicine because I realized that health is transcendental for man." (Kevin) "I want to do more for [marginalized] populations." (Bianca)	8%
Interest since childhood	"From when I was really small, I would pretend with my dad that I would cure him." (Amanda) "I liked pretending I was a doctor and all that." (Lucero)	8%

(continued)

TABLE 1   *(continued)*

Reason for Medical School	Exemplar Quotes	Percentage
Family pressures	"[My father] convinced me and so I decided to enter medicine." (Diana)	6%
Career test	"They did a survey to find out what we liked and what we didn't. I don't like mathematics, but I like biology." (Rosa)	6%
Medical role models	"I always liked [that doctora's] treatment of patients; liked how intelligent she is. . . . She played a big part in my decision. I don't have any doctor in the family, and she was an example to follow." (Ricardo)	6%
Alternative plans fell through	"I was diagnosed with renal insufficiency [which changed my plan]." (Diego)	3%

filters to keep out people lacking the qualities of good medicine. Doctor Contreras said he always asked his students why they studied medicine and claimed that he one time heard someone answer "because I like wearing white" along with other vague answers like "because my dad is a doctor," "because I like it," or because they would become wealthy. His voice rising in indignation, he said these vague comments would never carry trainees through the hard times of medicine. He cautioned the interns that "our vocation is hard. . . . To come [to the hospital] on December 31 and leave your family; don't forget that." Doctor Morales agreed, saying that in his experience only a few of the interns he met had a true vocation for medicine, that many were "no good," and so the internship was a way to filter out those without vocation or who lacked "empathy for learning." He added that these types of students usually realized their lack of interest during difficult shifts. He concluded that his generation "who were already halfway through our careers" were truly dedicated to the practice of medicine. Gesturing to the watch on his wrist he said, "It doesn't matter the hour or the baptism" or other family duties, he believed that doctors like him were there for their patients.

Upon entry, interns are rapidly absorbed by and made aware of the rigid hierarchy. The transition into the internship and its associated high workload, long hours, and new environment cause a significant amount of anxiety and stress (Ortiz-Acosta and Beltrán-Jiménez 2011; Reyes Carmona et al. 2017) and can also reinforce deeper societal inequalities based on gender, class, or race/color.

Trainees begin a series of "abasements, degradations, humiliations, and profanations" that systematically mortify the self (Goffman 1961, 14). Though interns enter the institution voluntarily, they are beholden to its rules and hierarchy and are expected to obey; they cannot leave the hospital premises without permission or enter certain spaces without the correct attire or attitude. The newness of the space itself can be intimidating (Consejo and Viesca-Treviño 2008; Harris 2014), especially having to learn which spaces they can enter and what specialized procedures they need to follow before entry (Salhi 2016). The internship is the first real initiation into the life of medicine, though it is certainly not the last.

Over the course of the ethnography, I asked each intern what his or her primary duties were. All of them emphasized that they were the first to see the patient and so their primary duty was paperwork: writing the patient progress notes, checking that patients' clinical histories were up to date, and ensuring all notes and forms (partograms, laboratory work, radiology images, etc.) were in the patient's chart and that doctors' signatures were on the forms. The paperwork could be overwhelming—as when Nicolás walked by me muttering, "I'm mixed up with so much paperwork [*Ya me hice pelotas con tanto papel*]." Evelyn exclaimed, "One time I had to do a clinical history, and I [didn't] fall asleep until 1:00 A.M." However, paperwork could "save your life" as Doctor Marco reminded the interns when they groaned at the amount of paperwork they had to do—having a record of everything they had done would be important if there was ever any issue with a patient. These medical histories are longer narratives about patients and their cases, written for a (potential) future audience (Good 1994). Doctora Duarte made the same entreaty, focusing on the obligation to narrate patients' clinical stories, telling the interns that their duty was to do a deep medical history even if it was a tiring task:

> We have found all sorts of things, surprised by what the history can tell us; you can't believe how [patients] can be that ignorant to do what they do. But the history is there to reflect that. . . . So each time you don't feel like it, think of it as a challenge to sit down and start from the [patient's] background and everything. . . . The more time passes and the more patients I see, the more convinced I am that one has to sit and spent an hour, *ni modo* [even if you don't want to], to do that history, okay? Don't forget.

Additional duties included patient intake, rounds with the doctors, presentation of clinical cases, and performance of procedures like suture removal, blood draws, or catheter insertion. A significant task was to serve as *instrumentistas* (scrub technicians), a job that was described by one intern as learning how to open the surgical packs and organizing and passing the instruments and other materials (soap, gloves, or antiseptic liquids) to the surgeon.[3] Interns also had to rapidly learn about sterile and nonsterile spaces to prevent contamination (and scolding).

One male intern stated with a chuckle that he had matured significantly over the internship: "I used to feel weird seeing blood or using a needle or seeing boobs. . . . But now I feel absolutely nothing." A female intern emphasized that she had become more independent and responsible because "it's about patients who deserve care. So, if we don't fulfill our obligations, we feel guilty that . . . maybe something happened to the patient because we didn't do it correctly." Though they didn't articulate it overtly, when interns spoke about their internship, they tended to describe a progression from mundane and basic care to more interesting and complex care, gaining with each step greater responsibility for patient welfare and deepening their cultivation of a medical self.

PRESENTING CLINICAL CASES

The interns' training ranged from self-directed participation in enskilment opportunities to formal teaching that primarily occurred in classes and in the presentation of clinical cases. These *casos clínicos* focus the trainees' medical gaze upon their patients, reconstructing them from people (subjects) to cases (objects) (Good and Good 1989). In the process of depersonalizing and objectifying their patients, doctors minimize the personal and social elements and focus on the physical, organic, and pathological. They learn to act like doctors in these settings (Luhrmann 2000).

Presentations at both hospitals took place in an auditorium large enough to accommodate not only the interns but also residents and doctors from different specialties. In chapter 2 I briefly described the clinical case of the female patient with pulmonary thrombosis, copresented by César and Doctora Duarte. When César began his PowerPoint presentation, he followed the clinical history in the patient's file, slowly unpacking the information, illustrating the profound way by which medicine trains practitioners to rethink what aspects of patients' lives are important (Good and Good 1989), "We have a female patient, fifty years old, married, of Christian religion, with unknown blood type and place of birth." He listed the patient's "pathological background" consisting of "frequent sudden dyspnea [trouble breathing] since last year, as well as maximum rates of cholesterol, triglycerides, and glucose. . . . For nonpathological personal antecedents, she mentions a trip [to the beach] three days before her admittance on December 31, . . . with a duration of three hours in a vehicle, which caused a pain in the left pelvic member." He then described her diet as "Type T," a medical narrative shorthand for tortas, tamales, tostadas, and tacos, and that she led a sedentary lifestyle. In her obstetric history he said that she suffered from metrorrhagia (abnormal uterine bleeding). She arrived in the ER "presenting with dyspnea [while doing] medium efforts, which progress to minimal efforts. She also presents vomiting [for] two days. The physical exploration uncovers vital signs with a pressure of 140/70, cardiac frequency of 104, respiratory of 24, temperature of 36.5° C, and weight of 75 kilos and height of 165 [centimeters]."

In this process of story-making (Good and Good 1989) César continued naming symptoms and signs as a means to reveal the diagnosis: "We found her conscious, focused, cooperative, anxious, with dehydrated skin and mucosa, presence of rapid and deep respiration, with a generalized vesicular breath, with no additional sounds; cardiac noises with good tone and intensity, with no additional murmurs." After providing more details, he turned to his intern peers and asked them to begin the differential diagnosis: "What labs would you start by requesting?" After dialoguing with the various responses given by the interns, César continued by saying that the diagnosis from the ER was either acute coronary syndrome or pulmonary thrombosis. The patient was then examined by specialists, which revealed the different opinions that specialists have within clinical narratives (Good and Good 1989). The obstetrician found a painful uterine fibroid of "approximately 18 × 10 centimeters" and suggested a total laparoscopic hysterectomy. The cardiologist kept her under observation in intermediate care and gave her fluids and several medications, which César quickly listed to his knowledgeable audience.

After César's introduction to the case, Doctora Duarte began to speak, providing more details on the tests performed (echocardiogram, computed tomography [CT] angiogram, etc.). She stood at the front of the room and described how when she was called to come in to the ER, "I was told, 'She has dyspnea,' and I said, 'Aha.' 'She has this age.' 'Aha.' I was on my way to [New Year's Eve] dinner, but when they told me, 'She has a cardiac frequency of 130' that was not good." Using a Socratic method, she alternated between explanations and asking the interns in the audience, "What therapeutic approach or plan do you give if she has all these risk factors? What would you do?" She grilled them when they did not know the answer, sharply telling them that this information had already been shared by César. Emilio replied that he would go the risk–benefit route, "I would go for an anticoagulant to treat the thrombosis; I think that would be a priority before treating the myomatosis [fibroids]. . . . I would later deal with the hemorrhage, given that the thrombosis would cause death in the short term."

After further discussing the case, Doctora Duarte told them, "Each of you must generate your own criteria. And that's what we did. . . . We would deal with the hemorrhage later. . . . Remember, [patients] who have an acute pulmonary thromboembolic event cannot be subjected to a surgical procedure at that time. We need something to safeguard and prevent the clots from leaving. . . . Don't forget that you can at least place a security device, and which is that device?" One of the interns replied, "The vena cava filter." Doctora Duarte said that experts can insert it in ten minutes, using X-rays, which was confirmed by one of the surgeons in the audience. This was the suggestion given to the patient. Recalling the patient's high cardiac frequency she said, "Remember, the first datum for pulmonary thrombosis was tachycardia [accelerated heartbeat]; it's the first thing you need to think about independent of anything." She continued explaining, "So, remember, thrombosis is a reflection of something."

She turned to the interns and asked, "Which of you recalls Virchow's Triad for thrombosis?" Almost 150 years ago, the German physician and anthropologist Rudolf Virchow described three factors critically important in the development of thrombosis (Watson, Shantsila, and Lip 2009). The interns called out each one: venous stasis (blood pooling in the veins due to poor valve function), blood hypercoagulation (prone to clotting), and endothelial lesion (vein damage). Doctora Duarte continued probing their knowledge, asking the interns who were sitting further back in the room, "Why would this patient have hypercoagulation?" One intern answered, "Could it be in the phlebitis [vein inflammation] that the patient presented?" Doctora Duarte answered, "Phlebitis could be one cause, but look for another one mentioned, I've just mentioned it, the causes in hypercoagulation in women." Another intern said, "The progesterone she was taking?" while a third and fourth said, "obesity" and "vitamin K." Doctora Duarte said, "All this was the picture, and it was very difficult not to think she had thrombosis, right? But there was one more detail. What had she done in the previous days?" One intern said, "Traveled." Doctora Duarte asked, "How long was she seated?" The intern replied, "Three hours." Emilio then added, "Doctora, I don't know if you remember, but when we did the evaluation right there in the ER, the patient mentioned that she had gone to Acapulco . . . and that there she had scuba-dived and descended between four and six meters below sea level. And that's why you told us that the changes in atmospheric pressure can also be related to the clinical case." Doctora Duarte agreed, "So with all that it was more than evident that she had thrombosis. What we didn't know or what we had to discard was whether that was accompanied or exacerbated by the pelvic mass."

According to Seth Holmes and Maya Ponte (2011), the purpose of narrating cases in medicine—whether in written form in a medical history or oral form in a caso clínico—is to discipline trainees to edit out information that is not relevant (such as, perhaps, why this patient liked scuba diving or eating particular foods, or whether her religious background, age, or marital situation had created a situation that complicated certain forms of medical care) in order to create a linear narrative with sequential, independent units that are meant to be solved. Doctora Duarte spent the last few minutes describing the physiology of the heart and valves pumping blood, and the way that pressure differences played a role. She said that if there was a heart failure, the blood would remain in the left ventricle "and it starts to be like in cartoons, like have you seen the ones where there's a hose, and the dog, cat, or whatever stand on it and it balloons out?" She said this would cause a global cardiac failure.

The case generated much discussion among the doctors in the audience, especially concerning the patient's family's decision to withdraw from the hospital and go home. One of the doctors always present at these events was Doctor Navarro, a kind and slightly pompous gray-haired doctor with a large nose that dominated his face. He urged the interns to think through a patient's diagnosis, especially because many arrived in the ER with a prior diagnosis: "Look at the diagnosis, go to your interns' manual, revise signs, symptoms, risk factors, laboratory exams, and write them in your medical notes. This creates the difference between a quality institution and one [that is not]." His words emphasize what Calabrese (2011) refers to as manualization—encoded in manuals, regulations, standardization, and other bureaucratic needs that overshadow good caregiving. Doctor Navarro then summarized what he thought were the primary points from the case, emphasizing once again the linear narrative encouraged in medicine: the good vision of the ER team, their ability to identify the priority, and their correct protocol toward identifying a diagnosis. He added with a laugh, dismissing the patient's personhood and focusing solely on problem solving a case,

> There were other economic or general cultural elements that prevented the patient having a better conclusion; who knows what happened to her! But the prognosis was certainly very bad. But what's interesting is this: how all the conditions add up to obtain a positive result. So, this teaches you that next year, the next months, when you are all working in a doctor's office you have to do . . . a clinical test, think about the illness, and channel it immediately. Of course, the possibility of having a CT angiogram is not present everywhere.

His belief was that epidemiology was important in understanding health care: "There are three substantial elements: time, place, and person. Always." This was a lofty ideal that might have suggested a concern for each patient's personhood and circumstances; however, because of the way medicine is structured, trainees are ultimately taught to ignore the social and economic circumstances of the patients because this information "would generate uncertainty as to the potential causes and treatments of the patient's problem within a medical framework" (Holmes and Ponte 2011, 172). Though in these cases the physicians urged the interns to elaborate and deepen their use of the information, what they transmit to the interns is that cultural and social background are irrelevant for care.

YOU HAVE TO SUFFER A LITTLE BIT: MANAGING OVERNIGHT SHIFTS

Though interns complained about many aspects of their internship, the one that claimed the bulk of their grievances was being on call (*estar de guardia*), which occurred every three days.[4] Shifts began at 7:00 A.M. and ended around 3:00 P.M., except for people who had a guardia that night. In that case, the guardia would normally be thirty-two hours long—from 7:00 A.M. on day one to 3:00 P.M. on day two. Even when they had completed a guardia, interns were expected to return to the hospital at 7:00 A.M. on day three to begin the ritualized cycle once again. In a series of marked highs and lows, interns would dread their upcoming guardia, would be exhausted while in the middle of it, and would be practically giddy with relief when they were done. Post-guardia interns usually looked bedraggled and bleary eyed, their face puffy from exhaustion and lack of sleep. As research has shown, sleep deprivation affects memory (Frenda and Fenn 2016), even increasing the production of false memories (Chatburn et al. 2017), which can have significant effect on doctors' ability to perform the core tasks of medicine.

I heard from several interns that a handful of hospitals in Mexico had modified their guardia schedules from every third day to every fourth day; as Ricardo from Hospital Piedad said, with a gleeful smile, "They will work no more than eight hours!" Despite guardias being such a dreaded part of training, when I asked physicians whether the hospital would ever change the shift structure, most of them scoffed, saying that immersive guardias were the *only* way for trainees to have lengthy contact with patients and become skilled. Doctor Morales considered the internship as a transformative period for medical trainees. He said, "We're against bullying" but if a hospital managed the internship well the guardias were key learning moments. He added that when the most committed interns finished their internship, they felt that they had not learned enough: "They say, 'Why can't it be one month more?'" I heard Doctor Contreras frequently repeat to the interns how his own guardia was every two days and that the generation above him was a "true internship"—in which they lived at the hospital all year— so the interns now should stop complaining. "Now we want everything *light;* we have things easy. That's a weakness in your current training. It was harder for us. . . . So you have to suffer a little bit. Life is hard, but if you put some effort in, it will be easy."

This friction between past and present forms of learning, the values and assumptions espoused, and the nostalgia attached to people's recollections of their training was reflected in a meme posted online by a Facebook blogger who goes by the name El Médico Amargado (The Embittered Doctor), which read, "When I was an intern, I didn't sleep; I quickly finished all my intakes; I did thousands of treatments; I attended births left and right; I inserted intravenous cannulas and catheters, subclavian and tenckhoffs; I didn't eat breakfast, lunch, or dinner; I examined aliens, protected the hospital, and performed Miracles . . . Oh, and I even had time to study."[5] The meme, jokingly attributed to attending physicians everywhere, unapologetically shows the hard, overwhelming, and interminable hospital work. It also rapidly ratchets up from the ordinary parts of practice to the extraordinary, hyperbolic, and ridiculous. In doing so it mocks the hierarchy's nostalgic views of medicine, greatly exaggerating their heroic and godlike abilities and demonstrating how they conveniently forget the hardships they experienced.

SPACES OF FAMILIARITY

Hospitals are spaces where rules are rigid and ways of doing things are often ritualized (Salhi 2016). Even the modern hospital is a conservative place; its rituals and routines tend to outlast their rationalization as science or care (Anderson 2009). By their structure and people's ways of being within them, hospitals are what Erving Goffman (1961) calls total institutions; that is, if we look at hospitals as places of work and clinical training, they contain like-minded people who interact together for extended periods of time and whose lives are structured by the institution's administrative goals and power structures, in this case of clinical training and medical caregiving. One of the central features of a total institution is the breakdown of the barriers separating the places where people sleep, play, and work. Medical trainees in these spaces become a cohort with similar duties, responsibilities, and expected schedules. In the liminal phase present in other initiation rituals described by Van Gennep (2010) and Turner (1967), and most recently Salhi (2016), interns learn to conform and not question the standard, taken-for-granted knowledge. Over time, medical training homogenizes and deindividualizes medical trainees, and trainees acquire the space's dominant culture and values of medicine (Beagan 2000).

In total institutions trainees are constantly judged, observed, corrected, and examined (Good 1994). Sometimes this homogenization is violent and abrupt, creating inequality regimes that create and sustain inequities within institutions (Masood 2019). For example, in a case I heard about, new surgical residents at the largest public hospital in Mexico were told that they had two hours to go home to get their belongings before being kept in the hospital for twenty-one days without leaving. This abuse was supposedly meant as a welcome, "so they would adapt to the hospital"; most likely it indicated to the trainees that their now-incarcerated bodies and time no longer belonged to them. It transmitted a culturally violent hierarchy of values, with trainees' bodies having no value except as labor. Within these settings conformity is gradual, wherein interns at first might be uncomfortable with something they witness, but when they see no one question these practices they accept them as normal, resolve the inconsistencies, identify with them, and might even perpetuate them (Beagan 2000). Medical students have to resolve their inner conflict between being a good medical student and a decent human being; as Claire Wendland (2010, 30) stated, the price of learning medicine can be one's soul.

Interns at both Hospital Piedad and Hospital Salud had the same guardia structure, but, because it was a private hospital, Piedad provided the interns with

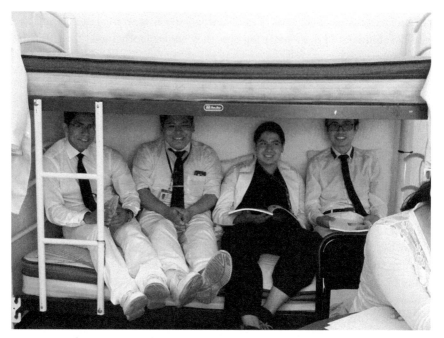

FIGURE 9. Male interns resting in the residence

a *Residencia* (a small resting room) where they spent their downtime and were sometimes able to sleep (figure 9). In addition to a locker room and a bathroom with showers, the residence consisted of one room with two bunkbeds, a table covered with laptops, papers, and other belongings surrounded by mismatched chairs, wall boards with notes, and a small wooden crucifix on the wall that had a Jesus figure inexplicably missing its limbs. Hooks by the door held stethoscopes and white coats.

The interns made the space theirs through personal belongings and photos, and used the boards for writing medical notes, jokes, or funny things they had said or experienced. On a high shelf sat someone's sneakers with a handwritten sign that read, "Danger, Code Gray, Noxious Gases." Someone's phone played Natalia Lafourcade's *"Nunca es Suficiente"* followed by "Hello" by Adele. On any given day I could find interns at the table, each on a laptop reading up on medical concepts or watching YouTube videos, while another sat on the bed putting on socks after a shower. Interns often slept two to a bunk, organizing themselves based on sleep (or snoring) patterns.

The Residencia was a space of familiarity where interns were more relaxed and where they could shed their performative medical self (by taking showers, contacting family and friends, playing music, or surfing the internet for comfort food recipes). They could simultaneously strengthen their deeper medical selves by studying cases and practicing skills. But they could do these without the stress from performing excellence in front of the physicians. Because it was backstage, it was also a space where they could complain and criticize the system or share a laugh about their training, as when Julieta complained to Samantha that one surgeon who had a reputation for never wanting interns in his surgery "scolded me once for having painted nails; he said they are a focus of infection." Samantha replied with a laugh, "You should have told him, 'It *would* be a focus if you would let me into [the surgery]!'"

Hospital Salud was not as well equipped. Bianca, an intern who entered medicine with the dream of providing medical care to rural, Indigenous, and marginalized communities, laughed ruefully and said "*Ya no dormí,* I didn't sleep" as she described how residences used to exist in the hospital basement, but they were converted into storerooms and now only the residents, but not the interns, had a small room for sleeping. She said, "We stay in the Emergency Room if the [beds] are not occupied, or we go up to Hospitalization to sleep. Any place. The nurses don't say anything to us. In other hospitals if they see you lying on a bed they'll say, like, "No! What if a patient arrives and you are here sleeping?' . . . But here they do let us sleep." One morning, when she was post-guardia, Bianca fell fast asleep on a gurney, her feet dangling off the bed; I could see the soles of her no-longer-sterile booties filthy with dried blood. Structurally, the spatial organization of a total institution like Hospital Salud, the lack of a place to rest, the shifts, and the value-laden expectation of having many patient-contact hours signals to the interns that they are meant to be working constantly, with no rest. The only recourse for interns at Hospital Salud was to learn to circumvent the structures, by finding hidden places to sleep or simply collapsing from exhaustion.

This issue of sleep went viral in 2015 in response to a thoughtless blog post that shamed sleeping trainees (Saul 2015). Doctors across Mexico responded in solidarity with the shamed doctors by posting photos of themselves in the hospital sleeping on gurneys, at desks, on chairs, or even on the floor with the hashtag #YoTambienMeDormí (I also fell asleep). Their posts showed how sleep was normal, how they circumvented the expectations, and how they sacrificed during their training, not only foregoing proper sleep but also sometimes food or hygiene. But, in their solidarity with their peers there was never any question about whether there was something wrong with a system that made doctors work this way (Castro and Villanueva Lozano 2018); the posts simply showed that this is what doctors *do.*

LEARNING ALONG THE WAY

Interns learned not only by doing and redoing their work and by presenting cases in front of attending doctors, but also by closely following physicians to learn specific forms of practice. When trainees engage in practice, they become enskiled while also signaling to their mentors their dedication to the craft (Gowlland 2019). Most mentorship in medicine is ubiquitous and haphazard (Rabow 2015), and trainees are exposed to both positive and negative examples of doctoring. Many doctors and residents were considered to be excellent mentors because they spent the time modeling good behavior and using positive reinforcement to make sure that interns learned properly. Others were disliked or feared because they were abusive or swore violently and humiliated interns who made mistakes during procedures. Gowlland (2019, 511) stated that "words, pointing and other gestures, demonstrations, eye contact" are all part of the mentor-student interactions. However, each doctor's communication style conveyed different modes of learning to the interns; those who used mimesis and created an environment conducive to bodily enskilment were considered to be better mentors. When I asked the interns to rank their experiences with different surgeons, Luisa from Hospital Piedad said that her favorite was a pediatric surgeon because "he explained with lots of patience about the clamps, the table, the patients. He would do it, and then I would do it." Her next favorite was an obstetrician "because I have to do it all myself. He would say it, and I would do it." The urological surgeon was fine "because he would do it alongside me. He opened all the materials and explained it all; 'You'll put this here and this there.' He explained everything." Her least favorite was an orthopedic surgeon because "he only told me, 'You will *instrumentar*.' I didn't know stuff about orthopedics; I could see files, drills, screws, but I didn't know about each one. [He] was very hurried, and we had a brief conflict. I got too stressed, and the nurse became the instrumentista."

Good mentorship is vital for a successful career. Mentors serve as role models, conduits of knowledge about practice and perspectives across the generations, and support systems for new members of the community trying to define their path. They can help to negotiate complex political environments, anticipate and navigate challenges, and facilitate networking (Turner, Bernstein, and Taylor 2018). Mentorship, akin to an apprenticeship, is embedded in ongoing practices and interactions and displays a tacit pedagogy (Gamble 2001) though it also demands explicit and active engagement by both parties (Paice, Heard, and Moss 2002). We should "conceptualize social interactions as being an integral part of the resulting technical skills, dispositions, and work ethics of the learner" (Gowlland 2019, 508).

Among the medical trainees I met, much of the technical skill was transferred in an explicit and mimetic manner, but attitudes, values, and approaches were more tacit, gradually assimilated through observation and direct mimicry. Trainees often imitate the intended actions even if they are not the exact actions of an expert (Gieser 2008). While mentorship might overtly focus on the transfer of a skill, there is also a wider transfer of associated attitudes and behaviors acquired from seeing mentors perform the inalienable property of the craft (Gamble 2001). In this process the interns acquired a medical self and learned to function within a moral economy of care (Higashi et al. 2013). This process is especially the case as medical students enter a clinical setting to be part of the institution and to fit in with its structure, rather than to fit the needs of the patients. As Anna Harris (2014) argued, they need to adjust in discursive and bodily ways to the new things, people, and ways of being; these adjustments are sensorial, including sound, smell, image, touch, and kinesthetic movement.

A frequent aphorism of biomedical training is "see one, do one, teach one." Among the Mexican interns I met, variants seemed to include "see one, study one, practice one" and "learn one, teach one." Julieta was in the second half of her internship at Hospital Piedad when we met. She was a quiet, but assertive, woman who dreamed of one day being an obstetrician who could help women have water births. She entered medicine because of her father's severe diabetes when she was a child, and she wanted to be a doctor to make sure that other people did not suffer the same thing—whether as patients or family members. She said that when she began the internship she just observed "how they did [procedures]." After this observation, she began to engage in practice, helped by the physician: "The doctor [would stand] behind me and teach me and tell me what was next, what I had to do, and then [I did these] on my own. [They] explain to you step-by-step; they don't just set you adrift." These "scaffolding techniques" create bodily proximity between expert and trainee (Gieser 2008), aiding in recall and embodied learning.

Iker best illustrated the scaffolded process of learning medicine. We met within a few days of the start of his internship at Hospital Salud, and he quickly became a good conversational partner and someone who was good to think with. Sporting a small beard and curly hair cropped short, Iker usually looked professional, dressed in pressed scrubs or in his whites (white button-down shirt, pants, shoes). He added a tie in a contrasting color, like the blue checked one he wore the day we met in the recovery ward of Salud's obstetrics and gynecology ward. He was an introspective intern who tended to see beyond the surface of his medical training. He said he had been drawn to medicine when, as a child, his mother became partially paralyzed and none of the doctors could figure out what was wrong, until one doctor who had been trained in Japan did a quick examination and resolved the issue with medications. From his childhood viewpoint, the doctor's care was miraculous and remained impressed upon his memory, prompting him to study medicine. He dreamed of being at Johns Hopkins one day, although he said that his English was rusty.

Iker was one of the few people who genuinely seemed intellectually interested in what I was doing there. During our first long interview we agreed to meet at the hospital's cafeteria, unimaginatively called "El Café del Sótano"—The Basement Café. I arrived early but avoided the food, as several people had warned me that it was known to cause upset stomachs. The smell of food was overpowering—permeating the rest of the hospital's basement, which also contained the ER, creating a disconcerting mixture of odors in a hospital setting: food mixed with suffering. Iker texted that he would arrive as soon as he could; he was busy in an obstetrics procedure.

When he arrived, we spoke about how he was managing the newness of the internship as well as how he was able to learn all the expected skills, names of tools and how to use them, and basic procedures. He chuckled and said, "Along the way. . . . I didn't even know the names of the surgical clamps too well." I was unsatisfied with this answer, especially because as an anthropologist my literal tool kit is quite unremarkable, consisting of notebooks, pens, and audio recorders, and my ability to wield these artifacts does not come at the expense of a patient's well-being. So I asked him more pointedly, "Okay. But how do they actually *teach* you? You say 'along the way,' but in what manner? Verbally, physically, they tell—?" Iker interrupted me and said, curtly, "Cellphone." Confused by the apparent non sequitur I stuttered, "What do you mean, 'Cellphone'?" He spoke forcibly, "Cellphone!" Pointing to his cellphone lying on the table he said, "'This is the cellphone; pass it to me!' . . . Like that."

Beginning to understand the process, I asked, "So that is how they do it? But what if you don't know the name of the clamp? I know the term for a cellphone, but if you don't know the name?" Iker explained more, saying that the process was exactly like that. He said that the surgeon would say the name of the required tool (for instance, "Kelly," a type of surgical clamp that resembles scissors) and that he might reply, "I don't know which the Kelly is." So the surgeon would touch his hand, point to the correct implement, and say, "Give me that one!" Iker sat back in his chair and said, "And like that, you learn it."

Of course, Iker provided a simplified and condensed version of the medical learning process. Not only are there hundreds of different tools, but many of them look exactly the same to the untrained eye. The physician Atul Gawande (2002) describes learning as a process that starts with floundering that becomes fragments, followed by knowledge, and "occasionally a moment of elegance" (22) wherein "conscious learning becomes unconscious knowledge" (21). Iker's narrative emphasizes this same process whereby the repetition of the haptic procedure of handling tools combined with verbally naming them reinforced his acquisition of knowledge, thereby shifting from what Rachel Prentice, in her ethnography of surgical education in the United States, calls "knowing that" to "knowing how" (2013, 114).

PRACTICE MAKES EXPERT

Instruments and the sensory skills needed to use the artifacts were a key part of practice, which allowed trainees to enact certain "doctorly" dispositions as they developed a medical self. Rice (2010) defined medical habitus as a conscious process in his examination of medical students mimicking doctors' use of a stethoscope as a symbol of doctorly dispositions. Habitus is transmitted through practice, which Bourdieu calls body *hexis* ([1977] 2000, 88), whereby people mimic individual and systematic bodily postures. A medical self incorporates bodily, sensorial, and self-making processes, such as how to navigate a medical space, how to exemplify expertise, how to embody medical institutions' unwritten and written guidelines for being a doctor, or how to act in a doctorly manner (usually perceived to be reasonable and common sense). A medical self simultaneously develops in the familiar and by new interactions and experiences (Harris 2014). As several scholars have shown (Rice 2010; Pink, Morgan, and Dainty 2014; Salhi 2016), some medical tools such as stethoscopes, clamps, cast saws, laboratory tests, gloves, or gel become visible symbols displaying a medical self and serve to enact the medical competence the trainees have (or aspire to have).

Figuring Out a Blood Draw

Yaretzi was a patient in Hospital Salud's emergency obstetrics ward who needed her blood drawn for some tests. As the newest intern, Wendy was assigned the task. A tall intern with a quiet affect, Wendy was well liked and respected by her peers. Her parents were enrolled in the public care offered by Hospital Salud, and she had chosen to do her internship there because she was familiar with the place. Sitting down on a chair, she wrapped a blue ligature on Yaretzi's upper arm and visually and manually checked for a vein. Evelyn, as the more senior intern, stood by her, overseeing her work. Petite, with slightly prominent teeth, long black hair that she tied in a bun on top of her head, and wearing big glasses in black frames, Evelyn was slightly awkward around others though she projected an air of efficiency, and she was always on the move—running samples, tending to patients, and talking to doctors and nurses.

When she saw no visible veins, Wendy moved the ligature lower, to Yaretzi's wrist, so she could check for veins on her hand. In the meantime, Evelyn unwrapped the syringe from its packet. Yaretzi looked away as the needle went in; she had tears in her eyes. When Wendy drew the needle back, not enough blood came out. Both Yaretzi and Wendy were evidently disappointed, and Evelyn's body language suggested impatience. Bypassing Wendy, as her junior intern, she turned to Yaretzi and asked, "Would you permit me to prick you once more? [*¿Me permite darle otro piquetito?*]" Yaretzi said yes, but looked frightened. Sitting down in Wendy's spot, Evelyn asked to see Yaretzi's hand, and, wrapping the ligature around her wrist, checked the back of Yaretzi's hand for veins. She asked Wendy to observe so she would know how to do the procedure properly. Wendy peered over Evelyn's shoulder, observing the procedure, and quietly chatted with Yaretzi. Evelyn prepared a second syringe, telling Yaretzi, "A small prick," as she put the needle in. But only a small amount of blood eked into the syringe. Evelyn looked disappointed, sighing deeply in frustration. She drew out the needle and taped cotton wool on the wound. As she discarded the syringe and needle, she called over an older nurse, using the title of "Miss" commonly used for nurses across all hospitals. Nurse Estela sat down in the chair, expertly tied the band at the top of Yaretzi's arm, swabbed her with alcohol, and swiftly pushed the needle in. The syringe filled up right away to Yaretzi's relief, who had already been pricked three times. Both Wendy and Evelyn look on, and thanked Nurse Estela for her help, both of them looking somewhat chastened by the nurse's obvious expertise. Wendy took the now-drawn tube of blood and marked it with Yaretzi's details in preparation for its examination in the laboratory.

Figuring Out a Cast Saw

A chubby, good-natured intern who took life in stride, Carlos was interning in Hospital Piedad's ER in 2014. One of the cases this day was Maricela, a four-year-old girl born with congenital hip deformities, who had a blue fiberglass body cast from her feet to her waist that had to be cut off before surgery that afternoon. The attending ER physician, Doctor Javier Gómez, a tall, balding, and bespectacled man, told Carlos that if he got the saw, he would show him how to cut the cast.

Holding the handheld saw, Carlos followed the doctor into Maricela's cubicle. No one explained my presence to the patient; with my white coat, it was assumed that I belonged. Maricela screamed when she saw us. Carlos paid no attention to her, and instead carefully observed the doctor swiftly cutting along the dotted line literally drawn along the cast's inseam. After doing one side fairly quickly, Doctor Gómez told Carlos to do the second side. Carlos took the saw and tentatively began to cut. Doctor Gómez left the cubicle to attend to other patients and did not stay to supervise. Carlos's inexperience was evident; he was much slower than Doctor Gómez, taking more than twice as long to cut. Little Maricela screamed the entire time. Carlos paused his cutting and told her, "Look, it doesn't hurt" as he touched the saw to his palm. Nurse Adriana looked on, checking that he did the procedure correctly, and handed him pincers to separate the halves of the cast. Doctor Gómez came back a while later and asked, "Done?" He stood at the foot of bed, overlooking Carlos and leaned over to check, telling him he had missed one spot, and then took the pincers and, with practiced hands, quickly opened up the cast along the inseam. The outside of the legs was next. Maricela screamed, whimpering, "It hurts, it hurts." Her mother held her and whispered, while her father stood nearby holding her foot. By now, I was struggling to hold back tears of empathy for Maricela; she was the same age as my daughter, and all I could imagine was the terror she must have been feeling.

Ignoring the pandemonium, Carlos continued slowly and carefully cutting without the doctor's supervision. Nurse Adriana stopped him and, pointing to the front of the saw, said, "You will have better control if you hold it from here." A while later Doctor Gómez re-entered and, seeing how little had been cut, told Carlos to let the saw cool down, later telling him to get another saw as "this one is going to *chamuscar* [burn out]." He told Maricela's parents that they would be in again soon. I followed them out, glad to briefly leave the terrified child. They rapidly attended to the other patients in the ER, checking X-rays, bandaging hurt limbs, and filling out paperwork. My back was hurting from hunching over my notebook and following the interns all day; I leaned against the wall and wrote field notes, trying to give my body a rest. It was at these moments when I clearly felt that being more than a decade and a half older than the interns placed me at a physical disadvantage.

Holding the new saw, Carlos seemed more certain of what he was doing and worked faster. "This one cuts better," he told the father happily over the loud buzzing of the saw and the whimpers of his patient. He carefully cut the lines along her waist, then picked up the pincers and tried to pry open the cast. Because the material was thicker, he had to alternate between sawing and trying to pry it open, resting the saw as it also threatened to overheat. Given that he eventually also had trouble using the second saw, one could conclude that it was not the saw that made a difference; practiced hands did. When this saw also became too hot to hold, he excused himself and exited the cubicle to find Doctor Gómez. He was immediately assigned to another case, that of a little boy with a hurt arm.

This pattern of Carlos sawing slowly on a screaming Maricela and then exiting the room only to be assigned to other cases repeated a couple more times. Each time Carlos entered the room, Maricela screamed and clung to her parents. He sawed with determination to try to get the cast open. By the time he did, all that was needed was to rebandage Maricela's hips and legs in preparation for surgery. Carlos could only find another attending doctor, Doctor Lorenzo Escobedo, a large, portly doctor with kind dark eyes behind glasses. He jovially greeted the parents and Maricela, "Oh, girlie! [*Ay, nenita!*] . . . I'm just going to bandage you like a mummy. Do you know what mummies are?" Maricela clung to her father's sweater as Doctor Escobedo swiftly bandaged one leg and then the other with Carlos's help. Her morning ordeal over, Maricela would soon be moved upstairs to the preoperative ward to prepare for her surgery.

Much of the learning and practice of the internship was about figuring out how to do things and then repeating them often until they became familiar—moving from Gawande's fragments to conscious knowledge. The aim is also for a state of unity between the user and the tool to create a fusion of two beings with one perception (Gieser 2008, 131). This was far from achieved by any of these three interns, who experienced failed scaffolding techniques and who still viewed the tools as separate from themselves rather than as an extension of the self. Each of these situations—Wendy's and Evelyn's failed blood draws and Carlos's sawing—exemplify the ways that interns learn the bulk of their skills from the ordinary encounters in hospitals. Despite these interns' lack of expertise or knowledge, the presence of these instruments, their medical uniforms, and the go-ahead from the attending physicians lent them a certain authority; that is, they were authorized to engage bodily with the patients and wield needles and saws (however inexpertly) that were not used by laypeople. On these days in question, neither ward was particularly busy; it seemed to be an opportunity for interns to learn new skills (or practice budding ones) without stress. It was curious, however, that Maricela's case was triaged: Carlos did not continually cut her cast, but a practiced physician did not cut it either, and no one continually supervised his cutting. Maricela seemed to be attended in between other patients, and her care was determined not by her screams, her fear, or her age but rather by the vagaries of an overheating saw.

How do medical trainees learn to *see* the body of their patient? Is this a process of seeing the whole, integrated patient in a broader biomedical complex? Or is this, as Janelle Taylor and Claire Wendland (2015) suggest, a process of "unseeing" and "unlearning"—learning to pay attention to the things, processes, and people that are "important" and simultaneously learning to ignore what is "not"? Like the casos clínicos I described earlier, trainees are encouraged in their interactions to be brief and direct and to ignore the extraneous (Holmes and Ponte 2011; Taylor and Wendland 2015). When Carlos focused on the saw cutting through his small patient's cast, was he unseeing her? His deep concentration on operating the instrument while only occasionally acknowledging Maricela, her emotions, or her parents seemed to suggest that was the case. The doctors never asked Maricela or her parents how they felt, and their social background or lived experience did not seem to factor into the way she was cared for. However, maybe the fact that it was Carlos's first time ever using a saw made him much more tentative and scared, so he concentrated more on doing it correctly. In Evelyn and Wendy's case, they each imperfectly performed the blood draw, pricking Yaretzi twice, but they seemed to know when to stop their practice and request help from an expert, in this case Nurse Estela.

One way to explain the disjoint between what medical trainees are formally taught and what they actually learn is the hidden curriculum (Hafferty 1998). Functioning at the level of organizational structure and culture, an institution's hidden curriculum is informal, multiple, ad hoc, and occurs during interactions outside of the classroom between doctors and trainees (Haidet and Teal 2015; Prentice 2013). A hidden curriculum is everywhere and is intertwined with all the practices in an institution so as to become invisible to those within the system (O'Donnell 2015). Within a hidden curriculum are embodied affects, judgments, and values within interactions (Prentice 2013). Taylor and Wendland (2015) suggest that "the hidden curriculum helps create the blind spots in which it then hides" (59)—that is, it hides in plain sight because its practices, like culture, are taken to be common sense and the way things are, like what happened with the casos clínicos described earlier.

The hidden curriculum is a powerful force that tacitly teaches people "how things work around here" (O'Donnell 2015, 7), communicating a message of what is actually valued, regardless of what is stated. The aspects that should be secondary (such as hierarchy, organizational structure, or technology) tend to be prioritized over cognition and learning (Morales-Gómez and Medina-Figueroa 2006) or over the screams and fear of a child. There is often a marked contrast between the idealized version of medicine that interns bring with them and the "contradictory and hard" (Consejo and Viesca-Treviño 2008, 17) reality with which they are frequently confronted. Jerald Kay (1990, 572) refers to this process as traumatic deidealization. For example, at the casos clínicos at both hospitals interns were reminded to be professionals—to behave according to the values of the institution. Trainees at Hospital Salud were scolded, "This is a clinical session; it's not a texting session." And yet there were frequent disjoints between the lofty values of a hospital's mission and the abusive or problematic behaviors enacted by physicians. The interns were repeatedly told that the interaction with the patient was key, yet the greater emphasis on bureaucracy, distilling information to the necessary pathologies, and paperwork suggested that their role was as typist, not clinician.

The term "professionalism" is used frequently in many professions, but it is rarely defined in concrete ways (Wear, Zarconi, and Garden 2015). Sometimes it simply refers to superficial and performative behaviors such as punctuality and appearance, which can be easily policed, rather than a deeper engagement with the values underpinning people's behaviors. Though most of the interns would be exhorted to behave professionally and to engage in practices that are considered an essential part of their patients' care, because of the hidden curriculum and what was left unsaid the values that they learned were that the patients' needs were not as important as their need to practice.

MAKING MISTAKES

Some interns were more critical of the ways that they had to transform book knowledge into bodily practice, especially of how they were taught by people who were barely more knowledgeable than they were. Nicolás was a second semester intern at Hospital Salud; during one interview we sat on an empty gurney in one of the wards in obstetrics and chatted about his thoughts regarding the internship. In most of our interactions he was reserved and not particularly introspective, though I saw him on several occasions making the residents roar with laughter at his physical or verbal imitations of other doctors in the hospital. He had entered medicine because both his parents were doctors and he had grown up in this sphere.

On this day, he spent a great deal of time telling me about his opinions regarding his issues with training, focusing on how he had learned to insert and remove different types of catheters. He said, "In my particular case I have found it hard to insert nasogastric tubes; it is one of the procedures that I find the hardest." Nasogastric catheter tubes are inserted through the nose into the stomach, and they are usually used for feeding or administering medication; their insertion requires skill and practice. Considering how ubiquitous catheters are in the medical care of patients in the hospital and how invasive and painful they can be, I was interested to hear his thoughts on learning how to manage them. He said, "In terms of the procedure, we learn from the [more advanced intern], the [one] with more experience. . . . He is the one who teaches us. [Then], when new [interns] arrive we teach them."

Perhaps because he been both the recipient and transmitter of this type of teaching, he was more critical. "I think that this has not really been the best way because we learn the wrong things that the [advanced intern] is doing. Because they don't even know if they are doing it well." He added with a chuckle, "That's how they were arbitrarily taught by some other person in an empirical way, who was taught by another, and we have not read the [proper] techniques." As noted by some scholars (Mankaka, Waeber, and Gachoud 2014), behaviors learned early are likely to persist. I asked whether anyone had corrected their procedures or checked whether they were done properly. He replied, "No, no one corrects [you], no one supervises [your procedures]. We do the work and done!" I continued questioning, "So there is no [resident] who comes and says, 'Oh no, you did that wrong' or 'Why are you placing it like that?'" Nicolás replied, "They don't supervise us when we carry out the procedures. But there are occasions when they realize that something is wrong, and then we do have to repeat [them]."

Interns described mistakes in varying ways, especially the response they received from doctors and what they personally learned from these situations. Wendy's harrowing experience during a birth is illustrative of how mistakes can have potentially catastrophic effects on patients' lives. As an intern in the obstetrics ward at Hospital Salud she was exposed to many clinical skills for the very first time. In one of our interviews she told me that she had attended her first vaginal birth the week before. "I had never attended anything before, nothing. And the baby practically came out on its own. Kind of like, 'Just catch it!'" While the baby's birth itself seemed to have been relatively easy, the complications for Wendy and her developing skills arose during the afterbirth (when the placenta emerges). She used a technique called a controlled cord traction (which is meant to be performed by a skilled birth attendant where traction is applied to the umbilical cord to draw out the placenta).[6] By any measure, Wendy was not skilled at this procedure. She said, "What happened was that I had never taken out a placenta before. . . . I added too much traction when I shouldn't, and I pulled out the cord and left the placenta inside." A cord rupture of this sort that causes a placenta to be retained in the uterus can be quite risky for the mother, potentially increasing her chances of postpartum hemorrhage (Urner, Zimmermann, and Krafft 2014), and it usually necessitates a manual removal of the placenta. This manual removal is considered an emergency procedure, which in private hospitals or those in higher income countries is usually performed under general or local anesthesia. Without anesthesia, as is the case in public hospitals in Mexico (because the limited quantity of anesthesia is reserved for cesarean deliveries and surgeries), it is very painful, consisting of a clinician inserting their hand into the uterine cavity and manually sweeping it to loosen and remove the placenta. Lydia Zacher Dixon (2015) elaborates on the routine use of this painful procedure during vaginal deliveries in many Mexican hospitals—even when the placenta itself is not retained. The postpartum examination of the uterus is a manual or instrumented exploration of the cavity to detect the presence of any placental (or fetal) remains and to check the integrity of the uterine walls (Camacho-Villarreal and Pérez-López 2013).

Wendy said she was shocked by what had happened, especially when Doctor Bruno, the junior resident said, "¡Ay! What did you do?!" She added that once the initial surprise had passed, both the junior and senior residents told her matter of fact, "Well, let's clean it up. . . . Let's get it out" manually. Wendy added casually that at this hospital the manual revision of the uterine cavity was routine, suggesting with her nonchalance that, regardless of her blunder, the outcome would have been the same for the patient. She laughed as she said she told herself, "Okay, I will not do *that* ever again!" She said that despite the mistake, neither of the two male residents scolded her, adding that Doctor Enrique, the senior resident who was guiding her on her manual skills (*que estaba metiendo mano conmigo*) told her, "Don't feel bad, just don't add traction." She concluded by saying that they told her, "It was good, considering it was your first time."

Charles Bosk (2003, 168) identified two types of errors in medicine: those that are more technical in nature and are a failure of correctly transforming theoretical into practical knowledge (which can be addressed through retraining), and those that are moral in nature, where practitioners fail to follow the ethical principles guiding the field. In his study he suggested that professional responses to each type of error are different—with superiors supporting those who make the former versus "degrading" or professionally excluding those who make the latter. Moral errors tend to be treated much more seriously in the profession because they "undercut the very fabric" of these professional relationships (Bosk 2003, 171). Wendy's mistake was a technical one, where she performed a procedure incorrectly but without the intent to harm. Gawande (2002) reminds us of the uncomfortable truth about medical training: we want perfection without our bodies being practiced upon. As patients we are often more comfortable with not knowing whose bodies are practiced upon in order for the doctor to learn. The patient who Wendy was attending was used as an object of practice so an intern could learn about birth techniques. The process of supervision during medical training is designed to mitigate harm to the patient (Gawande 2002). In this case, drastic harm was mitigated because both residents were working alongside Wendy, but the harm to the patient's body through the invasive and painful manual placental removal was unquestionable.

It is important to pay attention to whose bodies are practiced upon and whose are not—that is, the underlying structure of practice is a hierarchy of value and some bodies are more valued than others. Hospital Salud's patient base was primarily lower-income (which, as I described in the introduction, often intersects with color/race), and the hospital had many more trainees (residents and interns) whose purpose was to learn hands-on training on those patients. Conversely, Hospital Piedad's patient base was middle to upper income, and they usually had greater agency in determining whether their bodies were used for learning or in choosing to leave the hospital against doctors' orders.

What would an intern learn from Wendy's encounter? The formal curriculum would be the overt information shared, such as how to catch a baby, how to do a controlled cord traction properly, as well as the process of learning under supervision. They might also learn that they can count on their more experienced colleagues during difficulties and when they make technical mistakes. What else do interns learn through the hidden curriculum? Would interns learn that there are some procedures that can be practiced on certain types of patients and not others? Would they learn a hierarchy of value, wherein even if they are at the bottom of the hierarchy as interns, some patients are even lower? Wendy's admission about the routine nature of the painful manual removal of the placenta suggested that her mistake was a lesson about the value of patients and that a patient's health and well-being are less valuable than a trainee's need to learn.

NOT BASED ON MEDIOCRITY

Interns were repeatedly told by physicians, especially during casos clínicos, that they should carefully and thoughtfully work through the steps of diagnosis. Mauricio was a thin, bespectacled intern at Hospital Piedad who was always quick with a joke. During his case presentation, he made the mistake of "revealing" the patient's diagnosis (anemia caused by gastric cancer) too soon. He was swiftly interrupted by Doctora Jimena Aquino, a senior physician. "Wait a minute. Why don't you first do a clinical diagnosis? . . . Because the exercise should be for you to present the case . . . as if it were the first time this patient is seen. . . . Then suggest the diagnostic, laboratory, or anato-pathological studies, whatever is necessary, and then see if this coincides with what the patient had." Turning to the interns in the audience she said, "Otherwise none of you do a mental exercise to do the diagnosis. . . . So, it's very important [to share] the patient's personal pathological background or clinical history. And then we can all think along with what she might have, right? Because if you tell us everything, we don't think at all, right?"

The other doctors in the audience agreed and spent some time explaining to the interns that if patients came to the hospital for a second opinion it was "because the first one isn't working," so they should think of all these things once they were doctors. Interns were reminded that the internship was when they could ask questions, make mistakes, and say what they thought because they had experts alongside them to support and focus them. Doctor Morales said it was important for one to reflect "at what moment of any pathology's evolution could I have intervened and changed [the course of the disease]." He added that in his experience it was very different to see a patient in external consult compared with the ER because in the former a "patient brings to the surface all that might bother them" while in the latter "it was a specific concern that brought them" and doctors had to carry out a semiotic analysis of a patient's signs and symptoms. The doctors concluded by discussing that they should move beyond simply a "symptomatologic medicine," which only treated symptoms, to strategically investigate the cause. However, as noted by Nancy Scheper-Hughes and Margaret Lock (1987, 8), biomedicine has a "radically materialist" approach where doctors are taught to identify "the real (singular, usually organic) cause" of disease and rarely comprehend the "mindful causation of somatic states." Though the doctors spoke about patients' social and economic background, these were rarely articulated as causes of disease but more like factors to move past in their treatment.

As part of their training, interns were expected to hand over cases to their peers who had guardia. At Hospital Piedad these handovers occurred twice a day, at 7:00 A.M. when the shift began and at 2:00 P.M., when a shift was about to end (figure 10). The classroom where the handovers occurred was a long, narrow room packed with tablet desks facing a whiteboard with duties and the interns' names written on it and a metal teacher's desk on which sat a desktop computer and an unframed canvas print of a snowy mountain scene. The wall clock with a logo for a laboratory company was permanently stuck at 9:50. On one side of the room was a dark wood bookshelf with locked sliding-glass doors—behind which were standard medical texts in Spanish on obstetrics, pediatrics, hypertension, cardiology, internal medicine, and so on, as well as one large book on *Medicina Virreinal* (colonial medicine).

Handovers are routine in hospitals, where the care of patients is transferred from one shift to the next one. The information shared can include the patients' health status, medications prescribed, treatment plan, tests ordered, and evolving or resolving problems. Handovers should have both practical and pedagogical purposes (Wendland 2010), whereby trainees should read up on the cases to delve deeper into medical topics and answer questions through hypothetical extrapolations. Regina, a very driven intern whose determination tended to rub her peers the wrong way, strongly believed in the value of leadership during handovers; "so that there's discipline, there has to be someone to guide the [handover] . . . so they can teach . . . through example, and someone who knows how to *exigir* [to demand, to push someone to comply]." R. E. Klaber and C. F. Macdougall (2009) state that handovers can build the communication and analytical skills valued in medicine such as prioritizing, summarizing, presenting, and questioning—which, I would suggest, encourage interns to unsee by condensing the "important" information and leaving out the "unimportant" information about their patients.

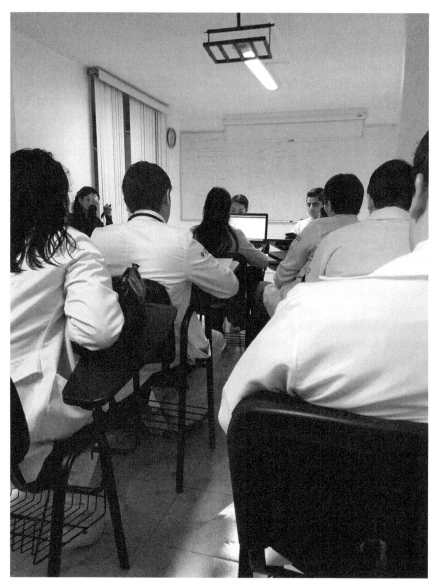

FIGURE 10. Interns from Hospital Piedad during a handover

The *entrega de guardia* at Hospital Piedad was primarily done by the interns with no regular guidance from residents or physicians, even though some interns like Regina had asked the directors to attend. This meant that the interns felt adrift. The interns concluded from this failure of mentorship that the doctors were not interested in this process. The interns at Piedad had internalized the perspective that handovers were a waste of time, and they had learned that these were just

something they were required to do that were used for attendance purposes—
they had to take a group selfie and send it to the director to show they were there.
Though some interns took handovers seriously, both medically and as a form of
becoming physicians, many regarded them as a brief downtime from their fast-
paced work, and they would nod off, check social media, or apply makeup.

The exception was one afternoon in 2016 when the anesthesiology residents
unexpectedly attended the handover, and the ensuing confrontation with the hierarchy exposed the existing interns' gaps in knowledge and practice. It also brought
to the surface some of the underlying assumptions about definitions of professionalism and medical practice.

The entrega de guardia had begun like all others, with all the interns sitting at
desks and one intern taking charge and listing the room number for each patient,
whose case was subsequently read out. A few minutes into the handover, Doctor
Maximilano, a senior anesthesiology resident, entered the room and sat at the
back. The interns quickly sat up, stopped rubbing their eyes and yawning, turned
off social media, and instead pretended they had been paying attention to their
colleagues all along. Doctor Maximiliano listened for a few brief minutes and
then interrupted them swiftly: "You need to take a photo of the medical indications and send it by WhatsApp. It's a handover, not a dictation and copying class."
He was soon joined by another resident, Doctora Mariana, who looked care-
worn, as though she was at the end of her guardia. She sat next to Doctor Maximiliano and immediately interrupted a female intern who was presenting a case;
she told her that the interns on call needed to present the case so they could get
to know the patient. She raised her voice and scolded them for being disorganized,
telling them their lack of professionalism was very disappointing. "It's not a game,"
she warned. Three more residents entered the room: Doctor Santiago, the chief
resident; Doctora Mayte, a young and friendly second-year resident; and the
newest resident, Doctor Juan, who was introduced to the interns and looked
somewhat nervous about his new job as a resident. Doctor Santiago told the
interns, "You do the handover to him in a formal manner. You have to hand over
the entire hospital to us. Get to know the patients. . . . You are doctors; you have
to control your own integrity."

When the introduction was over, Doctora Mariana asked the interns to explain
what a beta blocker was (which, broadly, are medications used for heart problems). It was a topic the residents had informally assigned the interns some weeks
before. It soon became apparent that the interns had not studied and had minimal knowledge about this class of medications. At first this irritated the residents,
who picked on each intern in turn and demanded they write the answers to their
questions on the whiteboard. The interns tried to cobble together knowledge,
which then was criticized and dismissed. "Too amorphous," said Doctora Mariana to one intern. "How do they work? On the heart? Adipose tissue? Divide it up
and write down the effects for each one," Doctor Maximiliano prodded another,

barking impatiently, "Explain it!" They berated each intern for his or her lack of knowledge or precision: "You should generate your own criteria. Generate questions if you don't know where to start."

Though the residents strongly urged the interns that part of learning was to generate questions, they did not demonstrate *how.* They asked Regina to write down ten different beta blocker drugs; with the help of her peers she managed to make a list of seven. When she was no longer able to add information, they scolded her: "You've had two months to learn this!" They then called up two interns and requested they write down how each drug acted, as many of them have different effects. Doctor Maximiliano rubbed his face in frustration and raised his voice: "You never studied the list we assigned. What the heck is the point of us coming to this handover if you don't study!? . . . If you don't know it, don't answer. Have you ever seen these medications on patient's indications? Have you never wondered about them? Medicine is logical."

Doctor Maximiliano tapped his suede shoe impatiently on the floor and proposed a hypothetical case to the interns for them to think about the effects of these drugs on the body. When they continued to answer incorrectly, Doctora Mariana snapped angrily, "You will give the patient tachycardia! You are giving them atropine?! You have just sent your patient to Saint Peter. They have destroyed her heart. These are human lives that we have in our hands! There is no wiping the slate clean." Doctor Maximiliano added scornfully, "You should have studied to be priests." Doctora Mariana continued, berating Aarón, a male intern, "How long have you been in the internship? You are too calm. You don't know anything. I would be scared of the [year of] social service." She added, "It's okay not to know," but she said the interns would be in trouble in their next career phase if they didn't improve. (A few days later, Doctor Santiago told me that sometimes the interns were even ignorant about basic medications—paracetamol or amoxicillin—and that he would sarcastically remind them, "Guys, [at the hospital] there are patients who, I swear, actually know what [these] are and how [they] work." He added it would be disgraceful for a patient to correct the doctor on this mistake.)

In this situation I suggest that there was a conflation between "information" (the facts and details about a topic) and "knowledge" (an analytical understanding of the information and being able to draw connections between it and the broader practices of the profession). Though on the one hand, the residents seemed to be assuring the interns that a lack of knowledge was acceptable, on the other hand they harangued them precisely because they lacked the expected information. They also spent much of the time telling the interns to practice medicine a certain way, but they never explicitly showed them how. The assumption was that in telling them, the interns would be able to transform the words into knowledge and bodily action.

Doctora Mariana paused and asked, "What do we call it when because of my fault or my error the patient dies?" One of the interns mumbled, "Iatrogenesis." Doctora Mariana said that all the examples and wrong answers the interns were providing were forms of iatrogenesis. Doctor Santiago, who had kept quiet for most of this time, simply observing his residents berate the interns, turned to an intern and said, "Would you like to cause iatrogenesis?" The residents reiterated their concern with these gaps in knowledge, stating that the internship was the time to correct any mistakes, that the interns needed to study more and be more responsible because they would soon be out in the world, treating real people. They said that interns should stop being mediocre secretaries, writing down medications and dosages, and instead learn and understand why medications were prescribed and what they did in the body.

By this time, the interns' affect was a combination of shock, despondency, and fear, as they pitifully tried to answer the questions, with each erroneous answer increasing the residents' displeasure. Several of them performed nervous movements; one intern squeaked his shoes on the chair while others moved their knees shakily from side to side. Doctor Maximiliano, still the angriest of the residents, harshly told the interns that, given the quality of their knowledge that day, they should just drop out of medical school and start a business as they were no good at medicine.

After more than an hour of berating and scolding, it was evident that the residents were still displeased and did not want to let the interns get away with what they perceived to be a lack of professionalism—the lack of knowledge combined with what they saw as a nonchalance toward medical practice. Perhaps in an effort to pacify the situation, Doctor Santiago turned to look at me writing notes and said, in reference to a conversation we had had a few days before where I had told him I thought the interns did a good job, "So that our guest doesn't think that we're the bad guys of the story . . . And like you have seen, the internship is many things, like my *compañeros* would agree." Looking at the interns he described what he perceived to be the tenets of a good internship:

> The internship is not just, "I come, I write my notes, I take down the patient to tomography, I go into the surgery late and waste time." . . . That is not the internship, guys, okay? The internship is the *last* phase to be formed as general practitioners. Like I've told you before, general practitioners that are good, and believe me, I've seen general practitioners who attend better than a specialist. But they are good general practitioners because *they* decided to be so. . . . They are not based on mediocrity. . . . The doctor who kills is neither the good doctor nor the bad doctor, because the good one resolves the situation; the bad ones know they are bad, and they decide to do [something else with their life]. The one who kills is the mediocre doctor because he says, "I *think* . . ."

He added that the slip came between the "I think" and the action, which, because it came from a guess from information rather than concrete knowledge, would be an incorrect and dangerous action where "your patient will die." He said, emphasizing a prevalent fear among doctors, "Maybe nothing happens, but death can also occur."

In his cautions to the interns he made use of narratives, particularly training tales (Pollock 1996) and parables (Stern 2015), that set up a binary between the good and the bad physician to instill a moral purpose in the interns. It also served to remind the interns of the prevailing fears among physicians—that they would not know what to do or that their actions would harm a patient. These stories, like those noted by Wendland (2010) among Malawian medical students, reference paths and routes through medicine, which are ascribed a moral value in which the doctors' own actions take part and can shape the broader trajectory.

Doctor Santiago made a distinction between the truly bad doctors—the monsters who purposefully harm their patients—and the "everyday bad doctors" (Gawande 2002, 89) who slip into bad medicine gradually, perhaps through carelessness, overwork, or ignorance. He bolstered his parable by referring to a clinical case discussed earlier that day about the death of a child where an attending physician had incorrectly prescribed aspirin for a fever, which had exacerbated an underlying condition. He drew from this training tale of medical failure to urge the interns to return to the accepted forms of medical practice and remind them of their responsibility toward the patients and the consequences of carelessness: "If you are the one who caused [this], there can be legal implications, and they'll ask you, 'If you knew that [these effects] could occur, why would you give that [medication] to the [patient]?'" Snapping his fingers for emphasis, Doctor Santiago said that if the interns did not have the basics "plus lots of common sense" they would kill a patient. In another physician's words from a caso clínico, "Now is when you can make mistakes. [Mistakes are] no longer allowed when you have a patient in your hands."

The residents stood up in preparation to leave the room, still very displeased with the interns. Before leaving, Doctor Santiago told the interns that he and Doctor Maximiliano were about to finish their residency and that they wanted to leave the interns with a message for their entry into the real world. Once again returning to a narrative style to encourage the moral development of their trainees, he said, "You never know when something will happen. . . . And if you are not ready, don't have the basics, nor even a little bit of common sense, God forbid something bad happens. So, please, study a lot. . . . It's not just about looking cool and hanging out with the attendings. . . . It's study, study, study, be active, be proactive, ask, rationalize, why, why, why, why, why. Okay?" Soon after this final plea and the dire picture of the interns' medical practice, the residents departed as a group, leaving the interns to pick up the pieces. The air in the room was thick with the interns' stress and anguish and the remaining anger of the residents.

I spoke with Doctor Santiago a few days later, and he said the interns had complained to the hospital directors. Despite this, he continued to believe in his message toward developing the medical self of the interns. He said, "I am not a taskmaster or someone who brings them here just for fun. . . . But they are doctors, will be doctors, and if they are truly convinced of their chosen profession that they are passionate about" then the interns needed to work hard and study because they would soon have the lives of others in their hands.

The deliberate and passive forces that exert profound pressure on the interns during their training allow them to develop a medical self. Their medical self incorporates habitus and techniques of the body, melding with artifacts and tools of the trade, using scaffolding techniques to mimic their mentors, presenting cases in front of physicians, (un)consciously incorporating the broader political economy and understanding of what to see/learn and what to unsee/unlearn in their journey through medical school. Trainees learn to focus their medical gaze on what medicine values; they learn to construct patients into objects of analysis and diagnosis. These are all part of the interns' process of attunement and selving. They learn not to question the taken-for-granted assumptions about concepts such as professionalism and common sense. They learn not to ask for explicit definitions of these terms because to do so would suggest that these are not, in fact, general common sense but rather particular to these places. They learn to believe that informal, ad hoc mentoring will teach them the needed skills of medicine. They learn that different bodies have different value, and they position themselves within this hierarchy of value in their practice. They learn to practice even when they are adrift.

4 · INTERNALIZING AND REPRODUCING VIOLENCE

It's true that the upper hierarchy is always managed by men. So that influences the way that the hospital interacts with women.

—Diana, intern at Hospital Piedad

You consider the moral part and that you shouldn't be doing [an unnecessary procedure], but, sadly, in the end, you do it. Because want to or not, it's part of how you are learning.... And, because of the hierarchies, you have no way to decide "if I do it or not" and they are ordering you to do it.

—Julieta, intern at Hospital Piedad

On September 8, 2017, Mara Castilla, a nineteen-year-old Puebla university student, disappeared. For days her distraught family and friends did not know what had happened to her. Her body was found a week later in an abandoned field outside the city. She had been murdered: abducted, raped, and strangled by the driver of the ride-sharing company she had taken after a night out at a party with friends. Mara was a victim of femicide, part of the much broader gender-based violence that is ravaging Mexico (Wright 2011; Haney 2012; Dixon 2015). Her death is, tragically, not the first nor last of its kind—the United Nations estimated that in 2016 at least seven women were killed every day in Mexico (UN Women 2017), with that rate increasing rapidly by 2017 to more than 3,000 annually (Jasso and González 2018).[1]

In the years before and since Mara's death, thousands of women have participated in protests around the country to demand that the government take action against the violence, fear, and harassment that women experience daily "just because they're women" (Camhaji and Barragán 2017). In a national survey, three out of five women stated that they had been victims of some form of violence in their lives (Riquer Fernández and Castro 2012). According to some sources, fewer than 10 percent of femicides are brought to justice (Camhaji and Barragán 2017). One of the primary underpinnings of this violence is the narco-violence that has swept the nation since the early 2000s.[2] Studies show that until 2007 the homicide rate was relatively low, with more than 90 percent of victims being male (Riquer Fernández and Castro 2012). In 2006, the state, headed by President Felipe Calderón, launched several military and police operations against the drug cartels with the aim of debilitating or destroying them. The plan failed, however, as the violence expanded in even more horrific ways, with the number of homicides skyrocketing to tens of thousands. The rate increasingly included women; in some regions, for instance, the risk of women dying by homicide increased 400 percent. The Mexican state responded to the violence with punitive measures, which privileged an increase in guns and police but did not address the root causes as the assumption was that the violence against women was individual rather than systemic (Riquer Fernández and Castro 2012).

Because femicides are pandemic, most of the female protesters who marched for Mara have participated in these protests multiple times; hashtags such as #SiMeMatan (#IfTheyKillMe) and #NiUnaMas/#NiUnaMenos (#NotOneMore/#NotOneLess) are used by women to show their resistance to and collective anger at the violence.[3] The hashtags have been used in resistance to the implication that the victims were at fault for their murders. As several writers have shown (Haney 2012; Rojas 2005; Wright 2011), many narratives from government leaders in Mexico have made clearly problematic distinctions between "good" women and "public" women (e.g., "slutty," women who work, etc.) to justify the deaths and assure people that if they knew where their daughters were there would be nothing to fear. Many of the political responses to women's voices have been to silence them (Rojas 2005). These protests are also an effort for women to be heard, to reclaim space, and to be able to live their life without fear of violence (Gottbrath 2017). For many, Mara's murder was the last straw, and it precipitated some of the largest marches against gender-based violence the country had seen (Gottbrath 2017; Nájar 2017).[4]

Gender-based violence is a structural phenomenon, built upon patriarchy, and is seen in private, institutional, and public spaces (Riquer Fernández and Castro 2012). Melissa Wright (2011, 709), in her deep analysis of femicides in Mexico, draws from Achille Mbembé's (2003) concept of necropolitics (the power, violence, and threat of death that a state wields as a technique of governance) to argue that the politics of gender and death go hand in hand when it comes to the gendering of space, violence, and subjectivity. As K. Eliza Williamson (2019) suggested, a tussle arises between biopolitics and necropolitics regarding women's place within society and the way that they are treated in medical spaces, particularly the hypervigilance and control of female/pregnant bodies on the one hand and the structures and their failure to keep women like Mara safe on the other.

The state of Puebla has one of the highest femicide rates in the country, with an almost twofold increase within one year: from 96 murders in 2016 to 141 in 2017 (Jasso and González 2018). A study showed that between 2005 and 2009 over 3,000 women disappeared in the state, almost 70 percent of whom were between thirteen and twenty-nine years of age (Pérez Oseguera and Espíndola Pérez 2015).[5] The neighboring state of Tlaxcala has a town infamous for being one of the most active organ and human trafficking hubs on the entire continent (Lakhani 2015). Nor is Mexico alone in gender-based violence; the UN estimates that one out of three women across the world has been a victim of gendered violence (a definition that includes femicides, child marriage, female genital mutilations, and other practices such as mistreatment of women during labor and delivery—known as obstetric violence).

What do these violent femicides have to do with medical training? Violent murders and the lives of female trainees might seem worlds apart, but whether women are female physicians, walking on the road, taking public transport, living their lives, or giving birth, the ways they are treated in Mexico are shaped by a much broader gender-based structure. Gender-based violence originates from this particular structure, where women are treated as though they are expendable. Women exist lower on the hierarchy, with fewer rights or recourses; their lives are shaped by targeted violence *because* they are women. Many women blame the macho culture of Mexico, where they were never free from fear. Gendered violence is never far from women's lives; like other women, interns, residents, and medical specialists have all been victims. Because these forms of violence are interwoven into the fabric of society, many of these women have also unwittingly become participants in this violence, perpetrating it on their female patients.

Using a scalar approach, in this chapter I link stories such as Mara's gender-based violent murder and the obstetric violence experienced in these hospital spaces by female patients to examine how harassment and the microaggressions I discussed in chapter 1 reflect intersecting, broader-level, gendered structures, particularly the messy ways that race, class, and color intersect and how they are amplified by gender. Even female doctors who have been victims of harassment internalize and reproduce inequalities based on gender, class, and color in their treatment of patients, which is part of the process of acquiring a medical self. All these forms of violence should be extraordinary—that is, happening rarely or not at all. Instead, because they happen so frequently, they have become an ordinary part of women's lives.

Obstetric violence is experienced by many female patients across Mexico and many other parts of the world (Castro and Erviti 2014; Diniz and Chacham 2004; Dixon 2020). This type of gender-based violence (Sadler et al. 2016) has been defined as mistreatment and abuse toward women during pregnancy and delivery, which could include any number of abuses, both physical and emotional (Savage and Castro 2017). Arachu Castro and Virginia Savage (2019) proposed six typologies of obstetric violence, which included verbal abuse (harsh/disrespectful language, patient blaming, public humiliation); poor rapport with women (including miscommunication of procedures and processes, language barriers); sociocultural discrimination (class, cultural insensitivity); physical abuse (unconsented or unnecessary procedures, hitting, uncomfortable touch, sexual abuse); failure to meet professional standards of care (delays, purposeful neglect, denial of medical attention, lack of supportive care); and health system conditions (failure to ensure privacy, lack of resources to provide more comfort to women, refusal to allow visitors or family members) (see also World Health Organization [WHO] 2015). As they argued, through these practices women lose control of their reproductive bodies.

Part of this violence is the reproduction of persistent historical patterns of societal inequalities (class, color, gender) within the clinical space (Davis 2019a), which value the reproduction of some populations over others, enacting forms of stratified reproduction (Colen 1995). Color consciousness deeply permeates the technologies of reproduction, and it structures how women experience their reproductive lives (Rapp 2019). A study by Roberto Castro and Sonia Frias (2019) calculated that within the past five years approximately one-third of women in Mexico experienced obstetric violence during childbirth. In these hospital spaces, physicians can be unwitting or deliberate perpetrators of this form of violence. Female practitioners are not exempt from perpetrating this violence. Sarah Rubin (2015), borrowing from Primo Levi's ([1986] 2017) concept of the gray zone, described in her work in South Africa an ambiguous space between the victims and perpetrators. That is, female interns and medical practitioners can be victims of gendered violence while also enacting it upon "their more vulnerable neighbors, sisters, and daughters" in medical spaces.

Recent work by medical anthropologists has drawn from a reproductive framework (Roberts 1997) to explore the intersections of race, racism, and reproduction and how racism functions as a mechanism "for the perpetuation *and* mediation of social inequality" (Valdez and Deomampo 2019, 556). They show how impoverished or racialized female patients must rely on substandard, under-resourced, or underfunded health care (Edu 2019). In these contexts the effect of temporal and architectural structures profoundly shapes the negative experiences of racialized patients (Andaya 2019). Narratives of health and responsible reproduction devalue the reproduction of darker bodies (Edu 2019), whereby medical care can reproduce social norms about gender and sexuality (Falu 2019) or enact discriminatory and violent treatment (Gálvez 2019), thereby deeply shaping birth outcomes (Davis 2019a). To counteract some of these structures, some patients are able to make use of technology to index their whiteness and inhabit their desired social position (Braff 2013; Roberts 2012).

Ultimately, what this analysis will show is the complexity behind the intersection of gender with Mexico's structural pigmentocracy and the impact of this intersection on medical practice. As Elise Andaya (2019) showed in her work in a public hospital in the United States, class and educational status can be just as important as race in creating difference. Rayna Rapp (2019) reminds us that the attitudes of clinicians are not neutral as they "enter into the construction of the very outcomes of discrimination that these professionals intend to explain and treat" (727). The identity that most impacts the interaction between female and male medical trainees is their gender—that is, the members of each group have similar socioeconomic backgrounds and social capital, but it is their gender that places women at a disadvantage. Similarly, the identity that most impacts the interactions between female trainees and their female patients is class/race/color, which Khiara Bridges (2011) has suggested is a "racial geography" (11), where mostly light-skinned clinicians provide care to mostly darker-skinned patients. Although both groups are female gendered, the female doctors are "above" the female patients because of their training and social background, shaping the power differential between them.

OBSTETRIC VIOLENCE IN HOSPITAL WARDS

Though female trainees can be (and are) victims of a broader form of gender-based violence, this violence can result in them also—sometimes unwittingly—becoming part of the violent system. One of the few interns who gave voice to the violence was Evelyn from Hospital Salud. One afternoon I invited her for a meal when she finished her shift, and we had a long conversation about medical lives during which she revealed some of her anxiety as well as her love for what she did. When we began discussing some of the doctors she had encountered, she described how, that very morning, she had witnessed a senior male obstetrician's interaction with a young patient. She said that this particular doctor sometimes made problematic comments to patients, and she described how he had examined a seventeen-year-old pregnant patient and performed a pelvic exam. When the patient complained of discomfort, the doctor told her, "It's just a finger; how then did you get pregnant?" Evelyn said that she was shocked by the comment and questioned the doctor right away. He dismissed her concern and mollified the patient by saying, "There, there, relax; you're pregnant, relax." Evelyn bristled at this situation, adding, "You can't treat her as if she was thirty or as if it was her second baby. She's young [chiquita]! I thought the patient would say something, but she left right after the consult." She concluded, "The tacto [pelvic exam] is already uncomfortable, and for [everyone] to see you [naked] and all, and those comments on top of that."

The transition into the clinical years is a central part of socialization when trainees begin to develop a medical self. A large part of what happens during medical training is that trainees learn to resolve inconsistent information and the discomfort it produces in them, learning to accept the inevitability of these problematic interactions. Evelyn had retained much of her discomfort at these situations, but many interns had gradually shed this discomfort and accepted these practices as the way things are. Through witnessing how male and female doctors interact, how "problematic" patient categories (young, rural, Indigenous, impoverished, and so on) are treated, how language is deployed to categorize and stereotype certain patients, or how much emphasis is placed on timeliness, paperwork, and following orders, trainees learn the hidden curriculum of what medicine actually values, as opposed to what it claims to value (Good 1995a).

Others have noted (Allahyari 1996) that people must wrestle with troubling moral issues as they create a new self. During their internship, when trainees engage in their first intense clinical training, they learn about the role of hierarchy, power dynamics, and interpersonal relationships in medical practice. They rapidly learn that some patients are worth more than others, that patients at public hospitals are treated rudely or not at all but private patients are treated with care. As Iker noted, how patients were treated depended on their physical appearance: "If they look, let's say, poorer, [clinicians] treat them worse, with greater distance, with sharper language, as if there was not much interest." As I mentioned in the introduction to the book, people in Mexico usually use class as a metaphor for race; Iker's use of the term "poorer" can be interpreted as "darker skinned" and lower on the whiteness pigmentocracy. Trainees internalize this value-laden system of which patients have value and which do not.

The care system for obstetrics patients in most hospitals in Mexico consists of a series of different spaces. Prenatal care takes place either at private doctors' offices or in *consulta externa* (external consults) in public hospitals. When patients begin labor (or they are scheduled for induction or cesarean delivery) they are often first attended in the hospital's emergency room (ER) or the obstetrics ER, where their intake is carried out, their medical history is checked, and they are also physically examined by the clinicians. In public hospitals the bulk of this work is carried out by trainees, while in private hospitals attending obstetricians take on more of this work (though not always).

The process of admission will be different in public and private hospitals. In a private hospital, patients wait in their private room until they are moved to the surgery and delivery ward, which is a sterile area where non-medical people (partners, etc.) are only allowed in by permission. In public hospitals patients are triaged. If they are not in need of immediate care, they wait in the ER area—which might have chairs or even beds for the patients. If they are in active labor, have an emergency, or are scheduled for a surgical procedure, they are moved from the ER into the sterile surgery and delivery ward (which is sometimes called *Tococirugía*). They enter alone, and are never accompanied by family members. It is routine in public hospitals for patients to receive intravenous Pitocin (an artificial form of the hormone oxytocin, which strengthens the intensity and frequency of contractions, usually making them more painful) and to labor on their backs lying on gurneys (Smith-Oka 2013a). In both hospital types, postpartum patients remain under observation for a few hours within the surgery and delivery ward, and they are then moved to their private rooms or shared wards in *Piso* (hospitalization) until they are discharged home by the hospital staff.

Ana's Birth

Ana was the private patient of obstetrician Doctor Leonardo García at Hospital Piedad. A light-skinned woman with a cheerful expression on her round face, she exuded comfort in this medical space. Her baby had been conceived through in vitro fertilization, at considerable cost, and she was very protective of her status—evidenced by the monthly ultrasounds she had received during her pregnancy. Research by Lara Braff (2013) on assisted reproductive technologies in Mexico connects race/color with access to the technology, particularly in the way that women claim greater whiteness and worthiness based on their fertility practices.

When Ana came into the hospital for her scheduled cesarean delivery, it was a slow Saturday morning, and the doctors were following a *futbol* game between two Spanish teams—Real Madrid and Rayo Vallecano. Emilio, one of the interns, was assigned to keep track of the game as well as perform Ana's intake. He had entered medicine because of his love of research, and he was eager to engage in research throughout his internship, proudly sharing that he was coauthoring two publications with one of the hospital's doctors. A man of few words, Emilio had a square jaw, large black eyes, brown skin, and a good-natured expression. He liked to contrast his white uniform with colored ties. He preferred the weekend shifts because interns would get more hands-on experiences than during the week. A natural leader, he took his duties seriously, taking on additional patients even if they were not his own. He had spent that morning in the hospitalization ward, helping physicians and nurses with discharging patients and was then sent to the ER to do Ana's intake. Emilio spent a few minutes carefully reading her chart so he would know her case and not ask the same questions: "Because first it's the [ER] nurses, then us [interns], then the attending doctor, and then the nurses in hospitalization, and even the anesthesiologist's assessment." He added, "one of my *compañeros* already completed this, and it's a vote of confidence for the patient when I know her name, what she's here for, and all that . . . At least that's what I believe."

I followed Emilio as he performed Ana's intake. She lay flat on her back on the bed in the curtained cubicle. She joked with Emilio as he asked her several questions to complete her chart—her diet, personal habits, family health, and details about her pregnancy, including contractions and fetal movement. He physically examined her—checking her heart with a stethoscope, checking the bag of intravenous fluids, examining her belly, and touching her ankle while asking if her feet had swollen. Emilio said that her baby's fetal heart rate was listed as 115 beats per minute.[6] When Ana expressed surprise, Emilio told her matter-of-factly that Doctor García had changed a few things in her chart to justify her cesarean delivery. She replied, nodding, "Ah yes, because of [my baby's size]." He said that after the cesarean delivery, her baby would be moved to an incubator for two to three hours so it would adapt to the extrauterine environment, while receiving heat and oxygen. She could choose to have *alojamiento conjunto*—rooming in—afterward if she wanted. She expressed pleasure at having her baby soon, although I found it surprising that she did not question the process of when she could reunite with her newborn. Emilio asked, "Will you get the aesthetic [incision]?" "Yes, please," she replied, as he told her that there were two incision types in a cesarean, "the normal [one] and the aesthetic," meaning a vertical abdominal incision for the former, and a low transverse one at the "bikini line" for the latter. The cesarean surgery was scheduled to begin at noon.

When we left Ana, I asked Emilio why it was a cesarean delivery. He replied, "Because her membranes have broken," there was possible fetal distress, and the contractions were not frequent enough. Doctor García was concerned that it could be another forty-eight hours before the baby was born if it was vaginal. Emilio added that doctors often changed details of the birth for privately insured patients so they would be covered, evidencing the economics behind unequal treatment.

At 11:45 I joined the medical team in getting ready—donning scrubs and sterile boots, facemask, and *panaderito* (baker's hat) hair cover—and crossing the sterile divide into the delivery ward. As one crosses the divide into the rectangular-shaped delivery ward, one finds the nurses' desk to the left followed by a set of glass doors leading out to hospitalization. Immediately to the right is the attending doctors' *sala de descanso* (resting room) and the postpartum area where patients are monitored before being sent to their private recovery rooms. Across from the nurses' desk is the whiteboard listing the day's procedures and the personnel assigned to them, and adjacent to these are the three surgical/delivery rooms and sinks for scrubbing in. At the far end is the storage room with medications and equipment used for obstetric and gynecological procedures. Although the equipment was the same as in public hospitals, everything was shinier and newer.

When Ana was rolled into the delivery room, the physicians introduced themselves to her. Her epidural was carefully performed by Doctor Helú, the chair of the anesthesiology department. In his late fifties, Doctor Helú was a tall and fit man with light skin, a craggy face, and beaked nose. Ana's husband was in the room, excitedly holding a cell phone to take photos of his wife and newborn. Although her arms were loosely strapped to her sides, Ana had a pillow to support her head, which was adjusted by Nurse Fernanda for greater comfort. Emilio was serving as second assistant to Doctor García—the attending obstetrician. Doctor García's corpulent body suggested strength but also gentleness; in his early forties, he had a small beard, his brown skin framed by large, brown-rimmed glasses. He gently washed Ana's abdomen with soap and then inserted a urinary catheter. Doctor Helú peered through his bifocals and asked Ana, "Does it hurt?" He then distracted her with questions about what she would name her baby and whether she was nervous.

Doctor García swabbed iodine on Ana's belly with gentle swipes with a small rolling sponge (like a roller used for painting walls). Once satisfied, he used a cauterizer to cut through the layers to reach the baby, using a transverse, aesthetic incision. The room smelled of charred skin. His first assistant spread the tissue apart, while Doctor García explained to Emilio what he was doing. Emphasizing risk, he said it was a cesarean delivery "because the baby is large; it weighs almost four kilos, and a vaginal birth is very dangerous." When the incision was large enough, Doctor García placed his hands into Ana and drew out her baby; Ana's husband dazedly took photos while Ana exclaimed over her newborn. The baby was rapidly taken by the pediatrics team to suction and clean. I could hear the repeated squelch of the suction. The baby (who weighed 3.53 kilos) was silent for several tense seconds, and then squealed loudly. The pediatrician placed the baby into the incubator; which Nurse Fernanda rolled out of the ward, toward the nursery. The placenta, umbilical cord, and blood-covered clamps were placed in a bowl away from the table.

Doctor García began carefully suturing Ana's incision, putting compresses into the wound and using the cauterizer to stanch the blood. As he worked, he explained the procedure to Emilio and allowed him to put in a couple of sutures. Doctor Helú explained to Ana why it would take more than 30 minutes to suture: "There are six, seven layers. . . . The baby comes out, the placenta, they clean the uterus so nothing yucky remains, and they suture you. You get a new package [body]." For the rest of the surgery the team and Ana joked about politics and the state of life in Puebla. When the surgery was done, the last details were left to the nurses and interns, who cleaned Ana's belly and vaginal region, bandaged her, covered her with a brown blanket, and placed her on a gurney to move her to her private room to recover.

Brenda's Birth

Though Piedad is a private hospital, it was founded as a maternity hospital for indigent women and has a foundation to serve them. Brenda was a young patient, not yet twenty, with brown skin and long black hair; her large belly was streaked with stretchmarks. She did not want a cesarean delivery. Her care was covered by the hospital's foundation, and so she paid nothing. Her family had come into the hospital with her, and they nervously stood by her bed as she was examined. It was an incredibly hot day, and there was little breeze flowing in the ward—I was sweltering in my white coat with sweat running down my back.

Brenda was attended by Doctor Elías Luna, an obstetrician/gynecologist, who was aided by additional medical staff, including Samantha as *instrumentista* to manage the surgical tools during surgery and Victoria as the pediatrics assistant. Samantha mentioned that it was a good opportunity to learn about birth because Doctor Luna was known as someone who "lets us do a lot [of procedures]" so interns could gain practice in medicine. A male intern told me with a chuckle that one could learn a lot from charity patients because the doctors let you attend to them in ways that they could not with private patients. Doctor Luna was in his late forties, and he wore thin glasses that rested on protruding ears, framed by his thinning hair. When I asked him how Brenda was, he said she would likely have a cesarean delivery. He had told her to take misoprostol—a medication used to start labor—at 2:00 A.M. in order to induce contractions, "but she didn't take it. . . . [Her cervix] is still hard."[7] Rolling his eyes, he said, "I think that she didn't take it until 5:00," adding before walking off that she was at 50 percent effacement (thinning of the cervix). Samantha said that Brenda was given misoprostol because she was "at thirty-nine weeks of gestation, and at thirty-eight weeks it is at term; so she was induced."

Throughout the morning, Brenda received several visits in her room from team members to examine her dilation, contractions, and fetal heart rate, with Doctor Luna offering to Samantha that he would let her do a pelvic examination so she could learn how to do it. Samantha mentioned to me that she was worried that the baby's heart rate had increased from 120 to 138, which meant that "the baby is very reactive, but [Brenda] doesn't have [good] contractions." At times Brenda looked nervous, chewing her lip in concern, while at other times, she gazed blankly at the television. Doctor Luna prescribed Pitocin to "have better and more productive contractions" adding that "labor hurts (*el trabajo de parto duele*)" but that she was almost at the end. Doctor Luna performed another pelvic examination to check her dilation, and told Brenda "your [cervix's] neck is very posterior; barely one [of my fingers] fits, and supposedly your contractions are now stronger." Turning to Brenda's young husband, he asked pointedly, "Did you actually note down the contractions?" The husband responded, "In the first hour, they were every four minutes, lasting thirty seconds." Doctor Luna spoke almost to himself, "They didn't last long," then he asked Brenda rhetorically, "What are we going to do with you?" Brenda looked at him in worry, her eyes wide with fear, her hands on her belly. He said he would return in fifteen to twenty minutes so Brenda could decide what to do. I asked him what he thought about Brenda's situation. He said, blaming Brenda, "It's just that sometimes the patients do what they like. You tell them one thing, and they do another. We gave her that medication at 11:00 P.M., and she says she took it at 2:00 A.M., but I think she took it at 5:00. So, from 5:00 to 7:00 there's been no progress. . . . We could wait for her all day, and then it could be tomorrow morning. But she also has low amniotic fluid, which worries us too."

I took a quick break to go to the bathroom—less than five minutes—and was shocked when I returned that in that short span the decision had been taken to perform a cesarean on Brenda. I quickly followed the interns into the changing room to don the sterile garb.

Brenda was rolled into the delivery room, and a female anesthesiology resident performed the epidural, gently chatting with Brenda about her hopes for her child and suggesting she get a transverse incision. Doctor Luna's male assistant was doing a pelvic examination to check Brenda's dilation—although it seemed unnecessary, given the cesarean surgery. Neither Brenda's mother nor husband were allowed into the delivery ward with her. She was lying uncovered in the middle of the room. Nurse Sofía was showing Samantha how to be instrumentista. Samantha admitted later that she was very nervous about being instrumentista and that she kept on forgetting the names for the tools. Victoria stood by the pediatrics station in preparation for the baby, keeping her gloved hands raised. Soft music in English was playing; the anesthesiologist asked Brenda, "Do you like it? Otherwise we can ask the doctor to change it."

When Doctor Luna came in, he covered Brenda with a cloth up to her neck while he prepared the space, telling her, "We'll cover you a bit." When he was fully gloved and gowned, he rubbed iodine on Brenda's belly, by dipping a gauze into a bowl of the liquid and rapidly swabbing her all over, bubbles trailing from the friction between skin and cloth. This was the same type of swabbing I observed in all cesarean deliveries and births in public hospitals. It is rougher than the roller used in Ana's cesarean surgery.

After the preparation, Doctor Luna began cutting Brenda's abdomen, using quick smooth cuts with a scalpel; spreading open the vertical incision, he dabbed it with gauze and then suctioned. He reached in and began to draw out the baby, with his assistant strongly pushing on Brenda's fundus (the top of her pregnant belly). The pediatrician looked over and asked, "It doesn't fit (through the incision)?" Eventually, Doctor Luna managed to take hold of one of the baby's arms and drew it out, placing him briefly on Brenda's belly, forgetting to tell her what the baby's sex was. The baby wailed as Samantha cut the umbilical cord, and Victoria wiped him down and weighed and measured him.

When teased by the team, Doctor Luna responded that he was not concerned with the baby's sex, and he turned back to the wound, drew out the placenta, and began to clean and suture Brenda's wound. The first few layers were performed by Doctor Luna and his assistant, and they chatted quietly about the process and why the baby had not fit through the incision. Victoria brought Brenda's baby boy over for her to see, all wrapped up in blankets; Brenda kissed him and gazed at him adoringly before Victoria wheeled him away in his incubator to the nursery. Victoria later mentioned that the attending pediatrician was very strict and wanted things his way, so when he was not looking she impudently wrinkled her nose at him.

Doctor Luna complained about the heat, and Nurse Sofía confirmed that the air was not flowing from the vents. Still intent on suturing, Doctor Luna asked Samantha for the suturing materials. He drew out one of Brenda's ovaries to show Samantha, who reached over to touch it. When all that was left was the skin layer, Doctor Luna passed the sutures to Samantha, and guided her hands, teaching her how to do a few of them. When the incision was sutured, Doctor Luna took an iodine- and merthiolate-soaked gauze and vigorously rubbed it all over Brenda's abdomen and vaginal area, as the other clinicians looked on. By now Brenda was completely naked, with her legs spread and her belly bright orange from the mixture of yellow iodine and red merthiolate.[8] Her arms were released from the straps, and she quickly folded them over her breasts. The team helped to bandage Brenda and place her on a gurney so she could be reunited with her baby.

The cesarean deliveries of Ana and Brenda reflected a classed and pigmentocratic hierarchy of value. Traces of moral hygiene perceptions are inscribed—sometimes literally—on patients' bodies. In both Ana's and Brenda's cesareans there were plenty of commonalities: they were both attended by male obstetricians, their arms were strapped to the side, they were unclothed, and they were cared for by kind and friendly anesthesiologists. Additionally, neither cesarean surgery seemed necessary, as the indicators were relative rather than absolute. That is, they resulted after a series of interventions (membranes breaking, labor induction) had an effect on the baby's heart rate and distress.[9]

Although neither of these births was particularly aggressive, they were shaped by each patient's social background, emphasizing racialized and classed stratified forms of care. They show the "subtle ways in which racist imaginaries are enveloped into institutions and practices" (Valdez and Deomampo 2019, 556). Although both cesareans took place in the same hospital, each woman had different social support: Ana had her husband in the room, but Brenda, despite being young, had no support. The type of incision performed was also significant: Ana's was transverse, as requested; Brenda's was vertical. Modes of medical care frequently extend historically rooted practices onto vulnerable bodies (Morales 2018; see also Colas 2017 and De López 2018). As Elizabeth Roberts (2012) described in Ecuador, scars from cesarean incisions bodily show a woman's ability to afford certain forms of care, whitening her body and differentiating it from the darker, poorer populations dependent on public care. Ana's and Brenda's incisions visibly instantiated their social and economic backgrounds.

Dána-Aín Davis (2019b) showed in her work on race and premature births in the United States that obstetric racism lies at the intersection of obstetric violence and racialized care, and it can have profound effects on maternal and child health and well-being. This is most visible in whose body is practiced upon. The bodies that are used for training usually belong to patients with less agency, created through an intersection of structural aspects like gender, skin color, and class. For instance, although Emilio helped Doctor García in Ana's birth, he only was allowed to insert a few sutures. Brenda's birth, however, was used to teach Samantha and other trainees how to examine dilation and suture skin; Brenda's ovaries were even brought out for display.

Although it is important for trainees to learn techniques and practices, the problem comes when only certain bodies are used for teaching and others are not, or when a race- and class-based "doubled discourse" (Briggs 2000, 247) classifies one group as able to tolerate more practice than other groups. In Mexico, social and economic differences are often mapped onto hospital types and spaces; as I described in the introduction, these frequently reflect the intertwining of class and color. Most of the trainees I spoke with over the course of my research told me that patients in public institutions or funded through charities in private hospitals had little to no choice about some of the medical procedures they underwent or the number (and experience level) of the people who could touch them.

TIMETABLES OF BIRTH

Like other scholars (Briceño Morales, Enciso Chaves, and Yepes Delgado 2018, 1313) I believe that neither medicine nor medical practitioners are inherently violent, but that obstetric violence emerges from the broader system, especially when a society's health-care system is discriminatory and "promotes inequality based on people's purchasing power." As Alyshia Gálvez (2019, 584) stated, the way government benefits are set up hierarchically racializes in a "virulent kind of structural violence" beneficiary populations as non-white and poor. That is, there is a stratification between patients who can afford to pay for private and better care and those beholden to the public system, who—because of a lack of resources, poor patient-to-physician ratios, or structural constraints—are more likely to be victims of mistreatment or abuse. This disparity was voiced by Julieta from Hospital Piedad:

> The difference [in care] is [based] on money. . . . It's very shocking to see the difference between a birth in a public hospital and a birth here. In a public hospital the [care] is very cold, . . . they remove the humanity, the beauty of someone being born, and the care. And it's really quite horrible; they treat them almost like cows, like "Okay, go, go, go!" I understand that there's a lot of work, but it's also not right the way they treat them. And here, well, [they have] music, video, and [it's] all emotional. . . . It could even be the same doctor that attends [in both places] and treats them differently.

The labor and birth of one patient at Hospital Salud illustrates some of the nuances of structural forms of violence present in these spaces and how the violence is "a systemic failure that reinforces outdated practices" (Dixon 2015, 449) and can emerge as an unintended consequence of people's enactment of medical protocols.

Miranda was in labor with her first baby. She was flat on her back on a labor gurney with candy-striped sheets, and she was connected to an intravenous drip with fluids and Pitocin. Even though Pitocin causes stronger and more painful contractions, Miranda was not provided any pain relief. Because of the lack of funds in the public hospital system, pain relief is a scarce resource that is usually reserved for cesarean deliveries. Doctor Marco, the first-year resident assigned to her case, had his hand on her belly, comforting her as she experienced a strong contraction. Funky electronic music played in the background.

The female attending obstetrician, Doctora Marisol Sandoval, walked over and quickly performed a pelvic examination, telling Miranda that she was fully dilated. Doctora Sandoval was professionally dressed in clean purple scrubs, her hair was gelled back into a ponytail, and her only concession to non-medical garb were her small diamond stud earrings. Her face was tight with a slight frown; she gave Miranda hurried instructions about pushing before walking off. Doctor Marco stayed by Miranda, explaining in a gentle voice how to breathe in, hold her breath, and use it to push. After checking her baby's fetal heart rate (the second time in under thirty minutes), Doctor Marco told Miranda that it sounded well but he would continue monitoring. He called over Bianca, one of the interns, and told her to stay with Miranda and time her contractions. Bianca sat down by Miranda; when Miranda got a sudden leg cramp, Bianca massaged her calf. She then told Miranda to push "like when you want to poop. It doesn't matter if you do [poop]." I stood by Miranda, massaging her and supporting her as best I could. She was tired—she had been told to push before her baby had descended and before she even had the urge to push; lying on her back was hard on her body, too.

About fifteen minutes later, Doctora Sandoval came back and again checked the fetal heart rate with a handheld Doppler ultrasound device. She told Miranda, "The [baby's] descent can last from two to three hours; it's normal." She added that if anything changed "we operate immediately." After doing another tacto (pelvic examination), she told Miranda all was fine, and that she would give her until noon before deciding on the following step. It was 11:00 A.M. She offered to sit Miranda up slightly, and told her to roll toward her left side. Bianca and I continued supporting Miranda through her next contractions.

Two more patients were rolled into the room, both of them scheduled for cesarean deliveries. By 11:15 Doctora Sandoval asked Doctor Marco and Bianca to check the fetal heart rate. Bianca placed gel on Miranda's belly and tried to find the heart rate with the Doppler, but was unsuccessful. Doctor Marco took the Doppler from her and found it right away. At 11:25 Doctor Bruno, a second-year resident, came over to Miranda. Grabbing one glove and some lubricant, he told her to lie flat on her back, "I'm going to examine you. It can be uncomfortable when I examine you, but you need to help me a bit. Take a breath." Putting the gloved fingers of his right hand into her and his left hand on her belly, he waited for a contraction. When Miranda contracted, Doctor Bruno told her, "Go number two, hard, hard, push, push below, push hard!" He told her he could feel her baby's hair with his fingers.

For a while, Miranda was left to labor quietly. Bianca and Nicolás, another intern, stood at the nurses' station filling out forms, which Doctor Marco checked, sometimes erasing their work and writing it anew. One of the other patients was rolled away for her cesarean surgery. I stayed by Miranda, supporting her through her contractions. A few minutes later Doctor Bruno came over to once again examine her baby's descent; he inserted his fingers into Miranda's vagina and told her to push hard. Doctora Sandoval walked over to inquire about the patient. Doctor Bruno still had his hand in Miranda's body, and Doctora Sandoval told her, "[Push] hard, *hija,* hard." Doctor Bruno told Doctora Sandoval that the baby was "right occiput transverse," which meant that the baby's face was pointed toward Miranda's left hip. This position is not always easy for birth, but it can be managed by a skilled attendant.[10] Amniotic fluid seeped from Miranda's vagina.

Getting a glove, Doctora Sandoval performed another tacto, inserting her right hand and keeping her left on Miranda's belly. Doctor Marco used the Doppler to check the fetal heart rate. He told Doctora Sandoval the rate; she nodded and told Miranda, "You're going to push really hard, all right? Your biggest effort. . . . Your push needs to last longer, *chaparrita* [honey]." At her next contraction, they both urged her "hard, hard, more, more, keep pushing, push, push!" Doctora Sandoval put her fingers in again, telling Doctor Bruno "It's not yet engaged." Doctor Bruno told Miranda, "We'll keep on waiting" and that she needed to push lower down in her body—"Don't keep it in the throat."[11] Both the doctor and resident walked away. Miranda had been two hours at full dilation, and the doctors felt she had not progressed enough. Doctor Bruno told her, "It's likely [the baby's] head doesn't fit."

The temporal tone of Miranda's labor changed; within a few minutes Doctora Sandoval returned and, without any preamble, told Miranda, "We're going to prepare everything to operate on you." She told Miranda she was fully dilated, but her contractions were not pushing the baby out. Doctora Sandoval rapidly listed the risks of a cesarean delivery, including the fact that because the baby was in Miranda's vaginal canal they would have to pull it back out, which could tear her uterus. She did not wait to see whether Miranda understood or had questions about this scary information. Despite these risks, it seemed they would proceed anyway. It was just before noon. Miranda was told by one of the interns, "You made a great effort, Señora Miranda; but we have to attend to the baby's health."

The slower, gentler pace of Miranda's labor abruptly became faster. The clinicians began to prepare her for the cesarean surgery: Doctor Marco placed her on her back and checked the fetal heart rate; a nurse rolled compression tights (to prevent clots) on her legs and then changed her bag of Pitocin for a bag of plain solution; another nurse came to shave her abdomen. Miranda continued with strong contractions. I sat down for a minute to write notes. I could hear Doctora Valentina on the phone asking someone on the other end permission to use one of the surgery rooms for Miranda's cesarean delivery. Doctor Marco appeared with several forms for Miranda to sign, and then sat down by Miranda on a low stool, using his phone to track the fetal heart rate while keeping his hand on her belly. He asked Nicolás to bring him Miranda's partogram paperwork. Doctora Valentina then asked Nicolás to take some papers to Doctor Arturo Casas—an attending obstetrician. He was in another area of the hospital, but the cesarean could not proceed without his signature. A male anesthesiology resident came over to Miranda to talk about the cesarean delivery and the anesthesia that would be used, asking several quick questions about her health.

After a few minutes, two residents and an intern began rolling Miranda's gurney out of the labor room and down the gray-tiled passages to the surgical rooms, toward Surgical Room 7. They had rolled Miranda halfway into the room when someone told them they needed to use Room 9 instead. The group stopped and Doctora Valentina said that they had requested Room 7; "Room 9 is not authorized; it can't be [in there]." A discussion broke out in the hallway, Miranda's legs poking out of the room, as the doctors discussed among themselves. When I asked what the issue was, Doctora Sandoval explained that, technically, the only room for cesarean deliveries was Room 10, but it was being used for another cesarean. Though it had a broken lamp, it was still functional. She said, "Room 9 is for births, but the table is no good"—it only had one position and could not be adjusted. She added that Room 7 only had one source of oxygen, which, when there are potentially two patients, could be dangerous. After some discussion, a consensus was reached to use Room 9, so they rolled Miranda out of Room 7 and left her in the passage across from Room 9. Entering the room, Doctor Marco, Doctor Bruno, and an intern detached the problematic table from the floor and dragged it out, leaving it desultorily in the hallway. The anesthesiology team went in right away and began setting up, even though there was no surgical table. Then the obstetrics team loudly rolled a heavy table from Room 7 down the long passage into Room 9.

The room was finally organized, and the team moved Miranda in, who shuffled over to the surgical table, which was rapidly set up with sterile drapes. Her lower quarters were fully uncovered, and the anesthesiology resident began to set up her epidural anesthesia. She was rolled onto her side and told to get into a fetal position. She whimpered with a contraction, and the anesthesiology resident told her in a kind voice that he would simply wash the area until her contraction passed. After that, her epidural was set up, she was rolled onto her back, and her arms were placed on boards perpendicular to her sides. Doctor Bruno opened Miranda's legs, and placed her knees to the side; using a gauze, Doctora Sandoval rubbed iodine on her belly, swabbing it everywhere, including Miranda's navel and vaginal area. Doctora Valentina inserted a urinary catheter.

I stood by the wall, next to Doctora Sandoval. She was the attending physician in charge and would be supervising Doctora Valentina who would serve as the primary surgeon, while Doctor Bruno would serve as first assistant. I could see his sterile boots coming undone at the back—his Nike shoe peeking out. Nicolás, as the intern, would serve as instrumentista. Doctora Valentina and Doctor

Bruno began the cesarean surgery, cutting through the skin with a vertical incision. Doctora Sandoval—not wearing a sterile gown—moved to stand behind Doctora Valentina. Nicolás passed the instruments hurriedly; he seemed nervous. Doctora Valentina placed her hand inside Miranda's body; there was a sudden gush of blood. Doctora Sandoval quickly put her hand inside too, and they drew the baby out. It was handed to the pediatrics team, and taken to the warmer for cleaning and measuring. On the way, a female pediatrics resident briefly showed Miranda her new baby.

The surgeons rapidly drew out the placenta; there was another gush of blood. Doctora Sandoval said sharply, "Get the suction, please!" Blood spattered on the floor, creating a large puddle by Doctora Valentina and spattering Nicolás and Doctor Bruno. Doctora Sandoval again stood behind Doctora Valentina, eventually dressing in surgical garb, which Doctor Marco helped her to tie. She replaced Doctora Valentina as the main surgeon; Doctora Valentina became the first assistant, and Doctor Bruno became the second assistant. Despite these several dramatic moments, there were no other issues, and the remainder of Miranda's birth proceeded uneventfully.

RITUALS, REGULARITY, AND TIMETABLES OF BIRTH

Miranda's birth resulted in the healthy delivery of her baby. However, despite this happy outcome, there was an undercurrent of obstetric violence. As Robbie Davis-Floyd (1994) argued, the baby is the most desirable end product of birth, with the mother being a "secondary by-product" (1127). There are similarities between Miranda's birth and those of some of the other women I have described—such as Brenda's cesarean delivery through the hospital's foundation where she did not receive the same degree of attention as Ana, the private patient. The violence in Miranda's birth was not overt; in fact, Miranda was mostly treated courteously. Doctor Marco was kind and considerate, as were the anesthesiology resident and Bianca.

The obstetric violence was instead more subtly threaded through some of the interactions, decisions, and structures, including at least four of Castro and Savage's six-item typology: blaming Miranda for not pushing properly (verbal), miscommunicating about the need for the procedures (poor rapport), unconsented—and possibly unnecessary—procedures (physical), and lack of pain relief or support from her family (health system conditions). Though pelvic examinations are a vital part of labor care, the World Health Organization has suggested that they should be limited to those that are strictly necessary and ideally done by the same provider (WHO 2018a). Not only are they uncomfortable, if they are done too frequently they can lead to avoidable complications such as an increased risk of infection. Miranda received many tactos by various people, sometimes in rapid succession. Only some of them seemed necessary to convey information about her baby's position or her dilation; others seemed to be done for training purposes.

There are additional complications when a human body is expected to behave in a mechanical manner and adhere to a timetable. When Miranda's cervix was fully dilated but her baby was not descending according to a biomedical timetable, the physicians' concern grew, which exacerbated the frequency of tactos and precipitated the decision to perform a cesarean delivery. Andaya (2019) stated that the temporal organization of obstetric care in biomedical settings privileges the time of clinicians over that of patients, resulting in an increase in interventions. Though the obstetricians were concerned about Miranda's baby's position, their emphasis on time structured their decisions, and they shifted from gently extolling her to breathe to rapidly preparing her for a cesarean delivery. Time became a factor in their decision (in the early requests for her to push, in the increased speed of tactos and interventions, and in the cesarean) rather than letting Miranda's body labor at its own pace.

Cesarean deliveries can be life-saving procedures, especially in cases where the mother's or baby's life is in danger. However, when they are used unnecessarily, they can transform from a neutral medical procedure into a violent intervention on a body. From my non-medical, anthropological perspective, Miranda's cesarean surgery seemed unnecessary. Though her baby's descent had "stalled," this was likely caused by a combination of factors: the baby's position itself (which could have been worked upon), her prone position, her inability to move around freely, the multiple people in surveillance of her labor, and the lack of familiar support.[12]

What makes doctors choose a riskier procedure, especially one where the baby had to be pulled from the vaginal canal? The decision to perform a cesarean seemed to directly contradict Doctora Sandoval's initial statement that a baby's normal descent can last a few hours. Those hours were not afforded to Miranda; she was forced to push before her body and baby were ready. Claire Wendland has noted that sometimes this type of fetal position resolves on its own, especially if the mother can move around.[13] Based upon the Doppler readings, Miranda's baby's heart rate was normal, and there was no indication of fetal distress. Doctora Sandoval's impatience with her progress seemed to accelerate with each tacto and each "failed" push, ultimately cascading into the decision to perform a cesarean delivery.

As a social and cultural system, biomedicine is structured around a set of rituals, beliefs, norms, and attitudes that shape its practice (Davis-Floyd 2003) and reproduce perceptions and ideologies about the value of people within the system. As noted by Robbie Davis-Floyd, these rituals also serve to give providers a sense of control over bodily processes they consider to be uncontrollable and risky. By performing rituals, people feel that they are "locked into" cosmic gears that will allow an individual to cross through risk and danger and emerge safely on the other side (Davis-Floyd 2003, 14). In her analysis of the complexity of so-called evidence-based practices in obstetrics, Wendland (2007, 225) has stated that two core values in obstetrics are safety and consumer ideology, both of which place primacy on technologies like the Doppler, the ultrasound, or the cesarean used by the doctors in Miranda's birth, located in the hospital and embodied by the doctors. In private births especially, these technologies, skills, and hospital space can be purchased to ensure the safety of a child, a choice not provided to women without purchasing power. Wendland (2007, 224) added that doctors' almost religious belief in technology explains why cesareans deliveries are becoming an unmarked category while vaginal births become increasingly marked as "unpredictable, uncontrolled, and therefore dangerous, appropriate for only a select few," as evidenced by the extremely high cesarean rates at Hospital Piedad, where some interns have never witnessed a vaginal birth.

The cesarean recedes into invisibility because it is so ordinary, while the vaginal birth is extraordinary because so much of it must be controlled. Wendland has argued that in these interactions the doctor's body is constructed as a site of safety because it controls the technology and the space. By contrast, a mother's natural body is a site of risk for herself, her fetus, and, I would argue, for society, too. From my anthropologist's perspective, subjecting Miranda to a cesarean seemed to be riskier than a vaginal birth; however, the doctors' reliance and belief in the balancing power of technology meant that, for them, the cesarean was the less risky choice. By telling Miranda that they must "attend to the baby's health," they were reminding her that birth was risky and tragedy could ensue, a process that "confers ritual authority" and "is used to keep dissenters in line" (Wendland 2007, 224).

Obstetricians are taught that labor occurs in a particular sequence of events that last a certain length of time. When a woman's body does not align with this mechanistic model, interventions might become more frequent (Davis-Floyd 1994). As Lydia Zacher Dixon (2015) noted, the issue of medical intervention in obstetrics is not just about medicalization but also about obstetric violence and human rights. Lupe, one of the female interns at Hospital Piedad, explained to me how she was taught to attend a birth at a public hospital where she had a brief rotation. She entered medicine because she wanted to help people. Her brown skin, black glossy hair, dark eyes, and expressive eyebrows were accentuated by silver-framed glasses and small gold earrings. Using her hands to emphasize her thoughts, she exuded kindness and compassion. When we first met, she was very nervous about practice, but over the course of her internship she grew in confidence as her enskilment became more apparent. At the very end of her internship she shared her knowledge about birth attendance, demonstrating her developing expertise.

Lupe said that it was standard for all patients entering the labor ward to receive an examination, including a tacto: "When the patient is . . . ten centimeters dilated, then you pass her into the [delivery] room. At that point the contractions are very regular. Each time the patient has a contraction you will tell her to push." Emphasizing the perception of temporal regularity within the biomedical birth model, she added, "The *producto* (the baby, product of gestation) emerges within approximately five to eight pushes." Using her hands to demonstrate the procedures she was taught, she explained, "With your left hand you hold the baby's head, to control the force with which it is expelled. . . . Once its head is out, you have to carry out the aspiration." Bending her left arm perpendicular to her body, she bodily demonstrated how to hold the baby, clamp its cord, and then pass it to the pediatrics team for care. Harkening back to the scheduled sequence of procedures expected within the biomedical model of birth, she continued,

> After this you manage the *alumbramiento,* which is the expulsion of the placenta. To protect the uterus you press upon the pubic symphysis, to make sure that only the placenta is coming out and there is no risk of uterine inversion.[14] When you have the placenta in the vaginal canal, you use your hand to turn the placenta so it comes out. You examine it to make sure it is complete, and that there are no sections missing. . . . Then there is a [manual] uterine examination to make sure that nothing remains, and to make sure there is no bleeding.

Dixon (2015) described this process as the manual scraping out of the uterus; her choice to use "scraping" encapsulates not only the visceral process but also the pain and violence embedded within the routine.[15] However, as Dixon noted a few years later in 2020, doctors were usually aware of the pain that this procedure could cause, but because they had been taught that this manual uterine examination was vital to prevent infection and they feared sending patients back home without examining them, they felt that the discomfort was worth the risk.

PERCEPTIONS OF *CULTURA*

Significantly, neither Miranda, Brenda, nor other racialized patients were consulted about the procedures they underwent, nor were they informed about their expected sequence. Miranda was simply told what would be done to her rather than being included in the conversation. She was never told why. As a patient in a public hospital, she had little agency. Even once the decision was made, she received hurried information—including the casually imparted information about the risk of uterine rupture. There was no opportunity for a dialogue, for her to ask questions, or for her to express her fears or desires.

Part of this lack of agency probably emerges from the perception that low-income patients lack *cultura,* so even if they have the information they would not make good choices. For instance, Doctor Luna assumed that Brenda was lying about when she took the medication he had prescribed, rather than blaming a failure in the medication or his prescribed medical approach. Doctor Roberto Burgos, from Hospital Piedad, told the audience at a *caso clínico*, "[I find it] strange that patients come to the hospital for care and don't even believe the doctors, right? [They say] 'No, you are crazy.' That's my issues with them, because of *costumbre* [local beliefs and customs] or whatever. But even in 2016 we have that issue regarding culture and beliefs and what have you." Emilio also blamed "the cultura of Mexicans" that made medical care more complicated because patients "wait until [they are] really sick to go to the doctor." He, like other medical personnel I met, commented that certain patients needed to gain more responsibility about their health as well as "life habits in terms of nutrition, exercise, [and] mentality." In our conversation Lupe stated,

> The patients have a low cultural level or, well, an educational level; they're skeptical and sometimes not cooperative. On many occasions, we received patients who'd had various babies. They are people of low income who don't want to *cuidarse* [protect themselves] with any family-planning method. And the reasons why they don't want to is because their *comadre* [fictive kinswoman] told her it doesn't work; because her comadre told her it hurt her; stuff like that. Not because they actually have a good reason for not *colocárselos* [getting contraception inserted]. But you can't force anyone to do anything. It's complex because you know you have criteria about what is best and sometimes patients won't accept it.

Colloquially, "cultura" in Mexico has a dual meaning, which embeds color/raced, classed, and gendered perceptions (Duncan 2018; Reyes-Foster 2018): either the presence of "problematic" beliefs and values among impoverished, rural, or Indigenous populations who refuse to change and become "modern" or the absence of "appropriate" values, understandings, and practices that align with those of mainstream and upwardly mobile Mexico. Contextually, impoverished, rural, Indigenous, and racialized populations are seen to have too much negative and not enough positive cultura. These "cultural" behaviors and practices are seen as obstacles to progress and are frequently blamed for why the country is the way it is. Wendland (2010), in her analysis of medicine's moral order, stated that culture is often seen as a problem to be overcome in order to provide medical care. As Whitney Duncan (2017) described in her work on mental health in the Mexican state of Oaxaca, cultura is considered to be a backward, insulated system that is transmitted through folklore and customs (like hearing information from *comadres*). As she shows, in these discourses the more "culture" a person has, the less capacity they are perceived to have to understand biomedicine and progress.

Culture becomes a marked category, inversely proportional to knowledge (and sense). Doctor Salmerón, a neonatologist at Hospital Salud, explained to the trainees that reproductive problems were not always about mistakes. Instead, "the problem is cultural. . . . What our population needs is information." Referring to the case of the baby born with gastroschisis (the intestines developing outside the body) which I mentioned in chapter 2, he said, "If this mother had received the adequate and timely information during her prenatal care, I think that maybe the problems might have been minimized. . . . But, at the end of the day, what's needed is cultura." He insisted that while prenatal education was important, care was not solely about including different nutritional components but "from the start one has to gather these people and give them this information; we need to provide informational talks to pregnant women." Though his words show concern with changing the broader attitude of patients toward well-being, his raced and classed statements assume that some patients are willfully ignorant or defiant of biomedical common sense, and that the only solution was to change patients' entire "culture" to make them value medicine.

This perception about patients' cultura was echoed by Victoria, who, like Lupe, was a kind and thoughtful intern at Piedad. In response to my question about whether she had ever witnessed any problematic interactions in obstetrics wards, she placed the blame on public hospital patients, explaining that "the only thing that bothered me was that there was no family planning, that they never had prenatal consults. . . . So, that was really stressful because you didn't know if [the baby] would be born well or not, if it would have any complication or not." Like Doctor Salmerón, she completely ignored structural and institutional issues that might have hampered patients' abilities to receive appropriate and timely medical care, stating that there had been some "complications with those babies. . . . For example, the baby dying because it was already dead from before. Or the baby having fetal suffering because they've only just come down from the mountain and it was the seventh child. . . . Or babies that were born at home and the mother would only come [to the hospital] so we could take out [her] placenta." Even though Lupe, Victoria, and other interns were very empathetic people who truly cared about their patients and worked hard at being both competent and caring, these beliefs about cultura and people's values are so deep-seated in Mexico that they become unconsciously threaded through most people's thoughts and actions. This hierarchy of value between private and public patients is a stratified moral regime between patients who can afford better care and impoverished "charity beneficiaries," who have limited options for care and might be treated as "favor beggars devoid of any rights" (Castro and Savage 2019, 124).

As Lupe stated, private and public hospitals are very different, especially regarding patient treatment and amount of work. Because of the higher number of patients in public hospitals, "you have more opportunity to do *manitas* (hands on practice). Because here [at a private hospital] we keep a certain distance in order to prevent troubles with patients." She elaborated on the ways that tactos were a central part of caring but also of teaching, clearly illustrating the race- and class-based forms of care: "[at Piedad] we don't do [vaginal tactos]; [in public hospitals] we do. You do it, the resident does it, your intern peers do it, as many times as needed. . . . Because there the patients will have vaginal births, and here the majority are programmed cesareans; so it's not that useful to do a tacto."

Lucero, another intern at Hospital Piedad, described a birth at the hospital that clearly showed how patients' agency differed. The labor sounded quite similar to Miranda's in some ways. She said that the private patient had been laboring for ten hours and had been stalled at nine centimeters dilation for approximately four of them: "She was almost [there], she just had a little bit [to go]. But the baby had not yet rotated well [and] was not descending well." Pausing, she added that the woman "had a lot of pain, she was very tired, and the anesthesiologist gave her pain medication, which caused the patient to stop dilating. So she ultimately had to be induced. . . . And the baby did finally rotate, but even then, the doctor used forceps." She described that though the husband was "hysterical" at seeing the forceps, the doctor was very experienced in their use. Chuckling, she said that the blame was on these private parents because "they were stubborn" about their request for it to be a vaginal birth "even though the doctor had told them it should be a cesarean." She concluded, "Though the baby was born vaginally . . . it was born with a large cephalohematoma [bruise] . . . with its cranium, like, with a bump."[16] Perhaps subconsciously guided by the moral regimes of care present in Mexican medicine where a patient's cultura determines doctors' degrees of disdain or exasperation, Lucero did not refer to these patients as ignorant or uncultured for not complying with the physician's mandate; instead she used the much kinder word "stubborn," which is very different from how a public patient might have been described under the circumstances. The label of uncultured suggests a permanent state only changed through education, while the label of stubbornness suggests a contextual state, disappearing once the situation ends. Despite the gentler epithet, however, Lucero's words index doctors as experts who know what is best.

As these stories show, obstetric violence is nuanced. In some cases, the abuse is unquestionable—like the unnecessary cesareans received by many (though not all) patients I met; like the racialized underpinnings of cesarean incisions, which resulted in Ana and Brenda, as private and public patients, respectively, having markedly different experiences and scars. In other cases, the obstetric violence was subtler. Most of the doctors were often simply trying to do the best they could for their patients under sometimes trying circumstances—not only the lack of sleep and the many patients but also the lack of infrastructure or supplies, such as all three of the surgical rooms in Hospital Salud having infrastructural issues (poor oxygen, beds, or lamps) that impeded good care. Questionable beliefs or practices sometimes emerged as unintended consequences of physicians' concerns with being (un)able to care for their patients.

The prevalent beliefs about cultura reflected beliefs about value that reinscribed long-standing discriminatory broader structures upon the bodies of patients. As Lupe concluded during our conversations, the treatment at private hospitals was better because patients paid for the care. Other patients, who had no purchasing power, learned to endure the care they received. However, they usually had to endure with much less information, much less knowledge, and almost no agency. As Castro and Savage (2019, 132) stated, women were usually resigned to the treatment they received and "to endure those issues alone, in the self-control mode they have been subjected to by the moral regime for the poor." Hence, "there can be no study of reproduction without an insistence on its constant renewal of racialization, racial privilege and racial discrimination" (Rapp 2019, 726).

I DON'T CRITICIZE THEM, BECAUSE IT'S VERY HARD

The forms of violence I have described here are not isolated examples performed by rogue perpetrators. I consider these to be the result of a much broader violence within the social structure (Briceño Morales, Enciso Chaves, and Yepes Delgado 2018; Jewkes and Penn-Kekana 2015). In a structure such as Mexico's, with horrific narco-violence and femicides, with violence within and outside clinical settings, and with women demanding to be taken seriously in professional spaces, is it any surprise that this violence is reproduced in obstetric spaces, where women are the sole patients? As Dixon (2015) stated, when "violence is seeping into people's homes" it is perhaps not surprising that it exists in obstetrics spaces, too.

Though some of the situations I have described might seem bleak, clinicians are generally doing the best they can for their patients in these spaces. As Samantha said after her experience rotating in obstetrics, "[It's] is very hard . . . and even more so in [public] hospitals because there are many patients. So one doesn't have the time nor the capacity to calmly endure a woman who's having her fifth child and is going crazy, [compared with] a woman who's having her first child and is doing super well, doesn't complain, says nothing. So, like, sometimes, well, that kind of despairs you. That's why, honestly, I don't criticize the [doctors], because it's very hard." Though she partially blamed the patients, she also acknowledged that the system itself was set up in a way that made medical care more difficult.

By taking a closer look at the medical education system, particularly its values, assumptions, and artifacts, we can also begin to understand how the hospital reproduces this violence. This is a system that emphasizes hierarchy (and the ensuing punishment, scolding, abuse, or discrimination) and creates an authoritarian system of values that is transmitted hierarchically (Castro 2014), eventually enacted on the most vulnerable: the patients. As Davis-Floyd (1994) stated, the culture of medicine emphasizes hierarchy and technology in birth, which results in a system that "technocratizes a natural process." In this way, doctors become the creators of the system "in the image we have chosen as [a] guiding metaphor."

The extraordinary effort female trainees expended to assert their legitimacy in this profession was often exhausting, demeaning, dehumanizing, and, at times, seemingly futile. This process generates an enduring hierarchy with men as superiors and women as subordinates. And yet, the identity of "woman doctor" can be especially conflictive and constantly shifting, where women have to erase femininity (but not too much) while also adopting masculine attributes (but not too many) in order to play the role of physician (Babaria et al. 2012). This situation prompts the question whether female doctors can be empathetic. Female doctors might become even more masculine and structured, eschewing empathy for control, sometimes even enacting violence on their patients in their drive to show how masculine they are and how much they belong. While there are no absolutes, women doctors have to tread a fine line between care/empathy, competence/control, and in/visibility.

"I think that if a woman one day entered a position of leadership," said Diana, "things could be different for women because then there would be someone who thinks like a woman." I want to conclude this chapter with Diana's words because they encompass all the tensions and frictions about women and hospital spaces. She said, "What we do need is teamwork, so like in the [upper] hierarchies you could have the brains of a man and of a woman working together. I think we would have better working conditions for both genders. There would be equity in saying, 'Hey, look, for women you have to be careful with this, this, and this.'" She added, "But it's very hard! Like, a director can't tell all his male employees, 'You have to be respectful to the women.' Because not all of them are going to listen to him." Instead Diana argued that these philosophies of how to treat others were part of people's upbringing. "Because, I mean, you could have ten women at the head of a hospital and harassment will continue anyway because those ten women are not going to show those adult men to respect women if they haven't learned it already. So it's something difficult to handle."

5 · THE BODY LEARNS
Transforming Skills and Practice in Obstetrics Wards

Never omit the physical exploration. Palpate their abdomen. The examination takes no more than three minutes. You cannot imagine how many patients I have helped by doing a clinical exploration.

—Doctor Leonardo García, Hospital Piedad

I think that the first fibroid diagnosis I ever did was in a purely clinical manner. —Doctor David Navarro, Hospital Piedad

They need to have the experience of [lots of] touching.

—Doctora Jimena Aquino, Hospital Piedad

Ultimately, the one who will [truly] teach you is the patient.

—Doctor Marco, obstetrics resident at Hospital Salud

It was nearing the end of a cesarean delivery at Hospital Salud. Doctor Arturo Casas was the attending obstetrician, guiding Doctor Marco, a first-year resident who was serving as the first assistant and was suturing the incision (figure 11). Senior residents handled harder cases, such as hysterectomies, so junior residents were assigned to cesarean deliveries, which were considered to be easier. Paola, an intern, was the *instrumentista,* a job that was a core part of all interns' training while in obstetrics. It is a grueling job that can be mentally exhausting, requiring an almost prescient understanding of the pace of the surgery. The baby had been born a few minutes before, wailing as it lay in the arms of the pediatrics intern. Another intern stood by the mother's head, phone in hand, asking her demographic questions, which were then typed into the phone to share with interns working in Piso—the hospitalization ward—where the patient would be sent after surgery. Doctor Casas joked with Paola as he blotted the incision. Paola gently bopped to the pop music playing on someone's phone, picked up a metal beaker, and poured some water on the incision. Doctor Casas

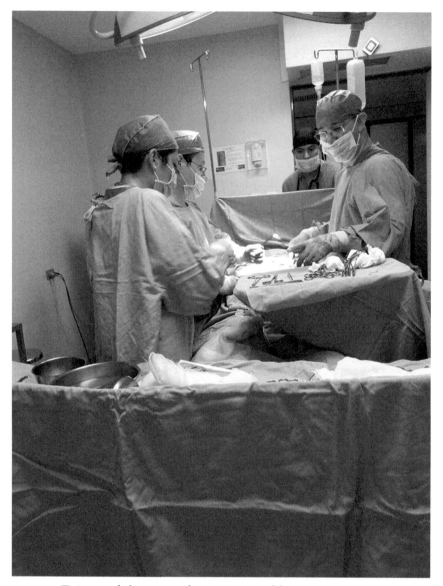

FIGURE 11. Trainees and obstetricians during a cesarean delivery

rubbed the wound and explained to Doctor Marco how to pull down the top skin and then to suture sideways.

Doctor Casas took a break and stood by me against the wall, trusting Doctor Marco to suture the next fatty layer. Knowing my interest in medical training, Doctor Casas joked that he was very good at scolding. Picking up a pair of surgical clamps, he pretended to hit Paola on the palm of her hands. Doctor Casas remarked that "she is not old school" because she did not even flinch. Paola laughed. She was known for her upbeat personality, easy smile, and cheerful Winnie-the-Pooh and flowered scrubs. All her peers respected her and regularly sought her out for advice.

Sitting down on a stool with a tired sigh, Doctor Casas commented that he had not performed a cesarean delivery in a while, as his residents did that work. A short man with dark brown skin and hair, he had a commanding presence and was quick to joke with those around him, though his affect could rapidly turn to displeasure. He wore dark-rimmed glasses, which he pushed back impatiently during procedures. He sat straight, leaned against the wall, and closed his eyes. Blood stained his gloves and gown. Doctor Marco continued suturing. He asked for clamps. Paola asked what type and then handed them over. Doctor Marco pulled half of the incision closed all at once. Doctor Casas rose, standing by Doctor Marco briefly. Seeming to decide that he was no longer needed in the surgery, he peeled off his gloves and gown and went to scrub his hands. Afterward he sat back down on the stool and scrolled through his phone.

Doctor Marco continued suturing, his facemask only partially covering his mouth. His nose and some of his beard were visible. While he seemed to be suturing well, the senior physicians noticed a mistake in his technique. Doctor Casas stood up and, with his hands on his hips, asked, "What are you doing, Marco?" The anesthesiologist joked, "Pass him the staples!" Doctor Casas replied, "Yeah, that's what I'm saying." The anesthesiologist scolded Doctor Marco on the placement of his sutures, "It's the other way around, *campeón* [champ]." Quickly correcting his mistake, Doctor Marco continued to painstakingly close the wound, peering carefully at both his hand and the thread as he sutured. When the incision was finally closed, Paola handed him some gauze. He requested scissors to cut the thread, knotting the ends of the sutures. Paola placed all the dirty instruments into a large metal dish. Doctor Marco blotted the sutures, aided by Paola who poured water onto a cloth in his hands. The anesthesiologist asked, "Are we done? All right! (¡*Sale!*)" and began to wrap up his materials so he could leave. His duties supervising his trainees over, Doctor Casas thanked the staff and walked out of the room.

The final steps of the cesarean surgery, primarily regarding the patient's care, continued and were managed by Doctor Marco, the interns, and the nurses. People's location in the prestige hierarchy (Hinze 1999) within this procedure were evident from their roles and duties, signaling forms of care and prestige. That is, active forms of care and practice are seen to be more masculine and prestigious, while more passive ones are seen to be less prestigious and more feminine. The most prestigious and central part of the procedure was notably senior and male, while the ending and less prestigious parts, involving more caregiving, were more junior and female, with the more senior and male participants peeling off after each phase.

The bloodstained drapes (*campos*) were removed. I could hear Frank Sinatra's "New York" playing in the background.[1] While the patient lay flat on her back, fully uncovered, Doctor Marco and Paola used gauze to clean the blood from her abdomen, legs, and vaginal area, placing a clean cloth bandage over her vertical abdominal wound. Paola put her hands on the patient's legs as Nurse Alma passed gauze to her. Though they attended to the patient's body as they worked, they talked past her, discussing the next cesarean delivery and how they must hurry to get ready. Doctor Marco asked Paola which intern would help during the next procedure. Paola replied hastily, "It's Evelyn's turn." Paola, Doctor Marco, and Nurse Alma held the patient and rolled her on her side so they could wipe down her back. After this, Doctor Marco stripped off his gloves and left the room to the female staff. The patient was moved onto a gurney where Nurse Alma and Paola bandaged her and dressed her in a fresh gown to cover her near nakedness. The pediatrics intern handed the patient her baby, before mother and child were rolled down the hall to the labor and recovery room. There, the other patients still in labor lay on their candy-striped sheets and exclaimed over the new mother and her baby.

At the transfer point lay a new patient on a gurney. Nurse Ofelia told me, matter-of-factly, "She is a stillbirth [*es un óbito*]."[2] Life coexists with death in obstetrics wards.

Ordinary medicine comes into sharp focus when compared to extraordinary situations like a stillbirth. As I will elaborate in the pages that follow, the ordinary and extraordinary facets of medicine are recurring themes. In obstetric medicine, the boundary between ordinary and extraordinary is not always clear. In the previous narrative, the cesarean delivery unfolded in a straightforward manner then was juxtaposed with the stillbirth, which was extraordinary for both practitioners and patients. And yet, sometimes, the extraordinary/ordinary binary is flipped—cesareans deliveries *should* be extraordinary, but they are so commonplace as to be ordinary. Vaginal births in these spaces are the exact opposite: they *should* be ordinary but are acutely extraordinary because, in some hospitals, they are extremely rare events. They have become performance opportunities for the practitioners, where gender and hierarchy are even more pronounced.

Embodied practice in these medical wards was always evident in the daily lives of interns and other medical trainees, as we can see from the previous vignette. The hierarchy was clear, with the two (male) attending physicians (the obstetrician and the anesthesiologist) in charge of the broader procedure, actively entering the body of the patient, and the trainees managing the minutiae: handling instruments, suturing, and patient care. Here the symbolic and embodied work of gender shapes the structure of medical practice (Hinze 1999). The bodies of the practitioners were evident in all these medical contexts as physical objects wielding tools or connecting bodies (patients and practitioners), as metaphors for these connections and interactions, and as metonyms standing in for the doctors themselves. The body of the patient is also visible as an object of practice rather than an object of care. In the vignette I purposefully depicted the scene as viewed from the medical perspective, with the patient at the center of the room but not centered as a person. This perspective shows the depersonalizing and medicalized way in which patients are often looked past (or through).

In this chapter I ask, What is the role of the medical body (that is, the body of medical personnel) as an object embedded within the clinical and diagnostic process? I answer this question by proposing that medical bodies are extensions of sociality, functioning as a tool for "somatic translation"—which elsewhere (Smith-Oka and Marshalla 2019) I have defined as the embodied process of learning, repeating, and making the body (both patient and physician) legible. In this chapter I focus on the ways by which medical bodies sense, feel, touch, and even smell in their quest for understanding the ills of their patients' bodies and how reproduction brings into sharp focus society's disappointments and desires. Like other anthropologists (Sharp 2000; Wendland 2007), I examine how bodies incorporate technology and become increasingly skilled and expert, becoming somewhat cyborg, a mixture of technological ability and flesh. That is, their "eyes [are] extended by ultrasound . . . their hands by scalpel and laparoscope, [and their] brain linked to databases of the latest clinical research" (Wendland 2007, 225). In my analysis I draw from the trainees' experiences in obstetrics wards: cesarean deliveries, vaginal births, and a stillborn baby.

HANDS TO TOUCH, HANDS TO SEE

Several key hospital ethnographies have examined biomedical spaces, and their authors added nuance to the development of the holistic medical self (Finkler 2001; Good 1995a; Luhrmann 2000; Prentice 2013; Street 2014; Wendland 2010). Furthering the arguments of these anthropologists I suggest that, as a tool of the trade, the medical body acts as a mediator, closing the social distance between practitioner and patient.

Hands are an obvious part of medical practice. It is hard to envision how a doctor can practice medicine without them. In such settings, hands are both the first and last points of contact between a patient and biomedical care. Of all the multiple body parts belonging to any given clinician, the hand is the one most in use in medical practice. It can connect and create distance, sometimes simultaneously. It is a perceptual instrument that senses while it acts (Anderson and Dietrich 2012), able to sense and see the "unseen problems in the suffering body" (Hinojosa 2002, 23). The hand connects the medical body with the patient, such as among Malawian medical students who learned through creativity and resourcefulness how to use their hands to detect twins, enlarged livers, or ruptured tubal pregnancies (Wendland 2010, 174). Alice Street (2014) borrows the term "anatomical geography" (92, citing Berg and Bowker 1997) to describe how looking, feeling, and writing reveal the hidden terrain under the skin and make it knowable. The act of medical practice is a fully embodied process.

The hand can cross boundaries as allowed through social scripts. It can wield technology and implements to cut, suture, examine, puncture, touch, or heal a patient body. Here I propose that hands, as the most basic technological implement available to clinicians, are at the root of medical knowledge. As anthropologists we can examine the role of hands, as extensions of the physician's body, to understand their function within the transmission of medical skills, knowledge, and attitudes within the halls of medicine. Physicians come to *know* their hands during their training, understanding them as extensions not only of their body but of the community and broader social structure as well.

Hands were the basic implements for the interns I met; they learned to use them as tools by shifting from theory (book knowledge) into practice (practical, skill-based knowledge). As Jean Lave and Etienne Wenger (1991, 32) pointed out in their analysis of situated learning, apprenticeships such as medical training are moments where people transform and become more complex and "full cultural-historical participants" in these spaces. Several interns told me that their hands were physically guided by their mentors during procedures so they could learn the motions and begin to internalize the knowledge. Once they gain mastery, the attention used in acquiring the techniques recedes (Csordas 1993).

Lucero, a cheerful and very competent intern at Hospital Piedad who had always planned to be a physician, described how she learned to suture. She said that one of the obstetricians taught her during surgery, "grasping my hands and explaining to me how to move my hand, how to take the thread, how to take the *pinzas* [clamps]." Interns stated that by moving their hands they learned the technique properly and that physicians step in "in case there is a complication with something, they help us, they move our hand, they guide us." By following the experts' movements, the trainees "feel into" a relationship. For this process to happen, their bodies must do the work without requiring them to be conscious of every movement they perform, gradually shifting from conscious attention to unconscious action (Gieser 2008, 312).

Doctor Marco, who I described at the start of this chapter, was one of the first-year obstetrics and gynecology residents at Hospital Salud. He was in his mid-twenties and sported a small, neat beard, which tended to look less neat the more hours he had been on his feet. He had the reputation of being slightly absent-minded and of forgetting his phone in odd places in the ward. He was a very kind and gentle physician, who treated both his mentees and his patients with respect. He was my first interlocutor to frame the idea of hands as a literal tool, alongside other medical tools such as sutures or stethoscopes: "Our tools are our hands; hence one always has to know, and it's what I have always told the interns, they have to know what their hand measures." He believed that knowing one's measurements directly translated to efficacy and practice when interacting with a patient. Physicians considered their hands as basic implements to treat ordinary cases but also as tools that they could use in extraordinary moments, such as bringing somebody back to life.

As a first-year resident Doctor Marco did most of the grunt work of residency life (following a patient's progress through labor and birth, filling out paperwork, and determining a patient's cervical dilation during labor). He was also expected to teach the interns, his immediate juniors, basic clinical skills such as history taking and physical examinations. His hands were simultaneously novice and expert—in the story at the beginning of the chapter he was a novice, learning the feel for a cesarean delivery but still guided by experts. He took part in the medical procedures, learning the techniques of the body (Mauss 1973, 70) and structural exercises (Bourdieu [1977] 2000) necessary for his chosen specialty of obstetrics. But when teaching the interns, his hands were those of an expert. He knew how to fill out forms, how to determine cervical dilation, how to use the handheld Doppler ultrasound to check the fetal heart rate. His hands were for teaching, too. The more active his hands became—and the greater their ability to enter into a patient's body—the higher he moved up the hierarchy of prestige.

In the obstetrics wards, patients in labor were cared for through a variety of ways—their fetus' heart rate was monitored through the use of handheld Dopplers, their contractions were timed, and, if they were expected to birth vaginally, their dilation was measured regularly through a pelvic examination. Pelvic exams are a vital practice to determine a patient's readiness to give birth, and they are considered both standard and necessary in modern biomedical care. As we saw in chapter 4, in Mexico a pelvic exam is called a *tacto*. Tacto translates to more than just "touch" (for which the Spanish verb would be *tocar*); its meaning conveys a more tactile element than simply touching. Tacto is about the *feel* of the tissue beneath one's fingers—its sponginess or hardness, its elasticity, its dilation.

Doctora Valentina, a third-year resident at Hospital Salud and Doctor Marco's supervisor, said that she learned to measure dilation by doing *tactos* in medical school using mannequins. She said, "We had these, like, cervical mannequins that [had] one [centimeter] dilation . . . six [centimeters] . . . and so you would put your hand in and then the doctors would ask you, 'What is the [dilation]?'" She said that later when she was in her internship, she became somewhat proficient at these tactos; her mentors showed her how to do them correctly on real patients. Although students learned to do a pelvic exam by first handling inanimate mannequins, in a hospital with a live patient the only way for them to do a tacto was by inserting their fingers into a patient's vagina and measuring her cervix by feeling through their hands (Smith-Oka 2013a; Valdez-Santiago et al. 2013). Hence Doctor Marco emphasized to the interns he was in charge of teaching the technique what they should know: "How long their hand is, how wide their hand is, and they have to know this when they open up [their hand]. Because after all, what for me might be seven centimeters, for someone [else] it could be eight, right? But the [interns] have to innately know what their hand measures." This measurement process was not idiosyncratic to Doctor Marco or to Hospital Salud but was practiced by other clinicians. Victoria, from Hospital Piedad, said, holding up her fingers and showing their dimensions, "Like this it is two centimeters, because my fingers are little. But there are fatter fingers where this is already three centimeters. But mine are like this; I would calculate this as two (centimeters)."[3]

What Doctor Marco argued was that a basic understanding of one's hands made them into better tools of measurement. In this process, physicians and medical trainees converted their nonstandard unit of measurement (their hands) into the standard units of measurement (centimeters) used in biomedical contexts across the world. I refer to this process of learning, repeating, and manually measuring as "somatic translation." Somatic translation is a way for physicians to read the patient's body with their own, making the body legible (theirs and their patients'). We can see this in action in the ways that the body in labor is measured, monitored, and timed repeatedly. This process equates the bodies of patients and physicians as they both become objects of measurement.

Thomas Csordas (1993) suggested in his work on somatic modes of attention that sensorial engagement is not about the body as an isolated object, but rather the body's situation within the world; this process involves attending "with" and attending "to" the body. Our body becomes a way to understand something about the world and the other bodies who surround ours. He proposes that the body becomes a sensorial means to engage with the world, attending to and with our bodies, attending to the bodies of others, and feeling others' attention to our bodies. This tactile attention (Sieler 2014) consists of the process of bringing the bodies of practitioner and patient into intimate contact, thereby developing what Anna Harris (2016) refers to as a resonating body, which allows practitioners to learn about others from their own bodies. We can expand on Brigitte Jordan's (1997) concept of authoritative knowledge to suggest that clinicians translate the measurement from the patient's body into written reports and charts that formalized what the patient *felt* into what the doctors *knew* about their body.

HACIENDO MANITAS

"Before you look at an image, you first have to touch the patient." One of the most significant hand-related metaphors in these hospitals was the notion of getting one's hands dirty, becoming handy in the process. The clinicians I interacted with referred to this as "*hacer manitas*" and "*meter mano.*"[4] These phrases are colloquialisms that imply becoming skilled by getting one's hands dirty, often literally. They are also used for more sexual innuendos, especially of groping and fooling around. Regardless of context, their meaning suggests the use of hands to familiarize one's self with another's body—whether a patient or a lover.

Interns defined meter mano and hacer manitas as gaining practice with basic skills ("Doing the practical work, putting in catheters, taking samples"), more complex skills (such as controlled cord tractions or manual uterine cavity revisions during a vaginal delivery), and physical contact with the patient ("hacer manitas [is] where you are allowed to *touch* the patient"). Only one intern eschewed the manitas expression, stating, "No, I don't like to [say manitas]; it's *practice*." From Doctor Marco's statement above about "hands as tools," we can unfurl the idea of what clinicians consider to be the tools of the trade, asking how these tools can become integral to their perceptions of medical-ness and in turn convey authority to those who do not know how to wield them.

Part of the process of meter mano was to train the hands to "see" a body. All senses come into play during medical procedures: clinicians' touch, sight, and smell intersect in their interaction with patients. Lupe, an intern at Hospital Piedad, reflected at the end of her internship about the process by which she had trained her hands to see the body of her patients through practice. Her language of competence became more complex as she advanced through her internship (Good and Good 1989), whereby she deepened her knowledge and became much more confident about her expertise and about becoming sensorially enskiled. She said, "When I say 'practice' I mean just that: to touch the patients . . . so you . . . move your hands properly, right? Sometimes you are afraid, you don't know if to touch or not to touch." She added, in reference to inserting an intravenous needle, "At first it's like having blind hands. You can't find the veins. And so 'hacer manitas' for me [means] that you try to insert once, you try twice, you try three times, and you start getting skilled with your hands, you more easily identify the structures that you have to know to carry out these procedures." She added that this repetition was also needed to understand and "see" radiological images, stating that "at first my eyes were blind." Through practice the interns learned to see structures where none was obvious (Good 1994, 74).

Learning sometimes entails a shift in the quality of one's engagement within practice (Gowlland 2019). Lupe shifted from using her eyes as a "disembodied, beam-like gaze" (Csordas 1993, 138) to a broader field of sensorial knowledge. She finished her story by describing the first time she touched a pregnant patient: "My *compañero* told me, 'This is a contraction.' I couldn't feel anything. But [afterward] I would touch [patients], and touch one and [then] another and another. And each time it was easier [to see]." For Lupe, blindness and an inability to see are about a lack of tangible, tactile knowledge about tissues and bodily structures. In her metaphor of sightedness she connects ideas of touch, expertise, sight, and knowledge into the idea of practice. Additionally, as proposed by Annmarie Mol (2003) and others, the act of seeing materially transforms what is being seen and how it is being seen. Bodies and their parts (fetuses, wombs, cervixes, etc.) in medicine are socially, culturally, and politically constructed; this process depends on who is doing this construction (Kilshaw 2017).

When people first learn a new skill, they are bound by rules, actively thinking through them (Dreyfus 1992). For interns, these rules might consist of asking *how* to touch, *where* to touch, in *what way* to touch, and where or when *not* to touch. For many, medical touch might feel invasive, whereby they get too close to another body (Good and Good 1989). By applying these rules and repeating their practice, interns begin to cultivate muscle memory, or what Csordas (1993) refers to as a rehearsal of bodily practice that is a "highly elaborated mode of attention" (139). Their bodies transform from novices to experts in a fluid continuum. They shift from seeing the body they are cutting or suturing to going more by feel and understanding of the way the body tissues are set up. That is, they go from seeing the body as a diffuse whole to feeling and understanding its component parts to once again understanding how these parts go together. The detailed attention to the rules and ways of doing dissolves into what Rachel Prentice (2005, citing Dreyfus 1992, 249) calls "muscular gestalt": ways that rules do not just dissolve into unconsciousness but become bodily fluid and flexible. Lupe asserted that only through repetition did she learn to "see" and understand the contractions of pregnant patients. In this process, stopping to think about the rules would erase the "smooth-flowing skilled bodily attunement" to the process and procedure (Rouse 2013, 252).

MANITAS AT PUBLIC AND PRIVATE HOSPITALS

The roles of manitas and learning, and the concomitant patient encounters, were differently experienced in public and private hospitals. As I have already mentioned, public hospitals in Mexico tend to be high volume: many patients, subpar infrastructure and equipment, overworked staff, and usually a multilayered staffing consisting of physicians, residents, interns, and nurses. In these spaces, the most marginalized rely on inferior, underfunded, and underresourced public care (Edu 2019). Private hospitals run the gamut of those that are large and well-funded, with a large staff and regular work hours, to those that are small and less well-funded, with questionable infrastructure and staff qualifications. Some of these private hospitals have the added layers of interns and residents, although not all of them do. Most, if not all, private hospitals have a low patient load.

The interns stated that in public hospitals they did manitas by engaging in duties that normally would be associated with the role of nurses, chemists, or orderlies. Most of them, however, emphasized that, while some of these "non-medical" duties were onerous, most of the opportunities for manitas gave them much needed (and desired) practice. Mauricio, from Hospital Piedad, said they learned procedures at these hospitals quickly: "They teach you two, three times and, *órale!* Go!" Some interns distinguished between the practice of public and private hospitals, such as one intern at Hospital Piedad who stated categorically, "Here one doesn't come to hacer manitas. We come here to *learn*." For him, learning skills was distinct from mindless repetition of techniques without knowing the "what," "how," or "why" behind them. For many trainees, there was a tension between practicing on a patient as an object of the medical gaze while simultaneously not seeing patients as subjects with agency.

While patient volume at public and private hospitals tended to be a factor determining how much access to practical experiences interns had, another important factor was the difference between patient agency at each type of hospital. As described by other scholars (Finkler 2001; Jewkes and Penn-Kekana 2015), patients in private hospitals tend to have greater agency—and the ability to say no to inexperienced interns practicing on them—than patients at public hospitals. Carmen, an intern at Hospital Salud, mentioned that she chose that hospital because it was "nice," with good infrastructure and a low patient load. She said she specifically did not choose a private hospital because "there are not many patients, and they don't let you meter mano, because in a private one the patients don't want that." An intern at Hospital Piedad added, "In public hospitals sometimes cases go there that you will never see in your life, and in the private ones you probably have less opportunity to do that. But they both have their pros and cons. In the private ones you can read, you can continue studying and preparing for . . . the residency exam. And in the public ones you can hacer manitas."

Putting her finger on the crux of the issue embedded in patient care in public and private hospitals, Julieta from Hospital Piedad, in reference to public hospitals, explained, "I don't know if it is just a bad habit or the fact of believing that because it's a public [hospital] you can do what you like. And the patients don't demand their right to complain. So they think that that is what they have to [put up with] and . . . I mean, when would you see a patient in a private hospital allow that?" She continued, "It is a problem from both parties: one that doesn't speak up and the other that thinks that they can do what they like just because it is public."

The concept of meter mano was not only from interns' and learners' point of view. Physicians saw the necessity of being hands on, of being clinical, as a central part of the process of medical selving. Doctor Elías Luna was an obstetrician/gynecologist I met at Hospital Piedad who I described in chapter 4. He held two jobs in order to financially make ends meet: one at Piedad managing the births attended through the hospital's charity foundation and the second at a high-volume public hospital in the city. He said that before interns left for their year of social service they should know how to "attend a birth, do an episiotomy, repair it. They need to know how to begin treatments of *all* pathologies. To know what it is. . . . They also need to know how we attend [a birth], and we let them do it little by little. Here it is difficult for them to meter mano. In teaching hospitals they are told 'you figure it out.' The problem is that this is both a teaching *and* a private hospital. The workload is very scant compared to [public ones]."

STILLBIRTH: LIFE AND DEATH IN THE OBSTETRICS WARD

I spent much of my time in these hospitals shadowing different interns such as Evelyn, Iker, Carmen, or Paola from Hospital Salud, observing their interactions and their practice. Their time in the obstetrics and delivery ward alternated between examining patients and handling the patient files in the *Cuarto de Médicos,* the Doctor's Room. I was shadowing the interns on the morning that María, who had had a stillbirth, arrived. Doctora Valentina was the senior resident in charge, delegating some of the care of that day's patients to Doctor Marco as junior resident, and to Paola, Carmen, and Evelyn, the interns. She was the only physician who wore a reusable surgeon's cap, which had a design of multicolored cats on it. Like most of the residents, Doctora Valentina eked out a living from the meager funds provided by the hospital residency combined with financial help from her family. Her scrubs reflected her penury, as she alternated between two pairs that were patched and torn in places.

Evelyn stood at the desk in the doctor's room, sorting the files for four patients. Our interviews occurred after-hours and in places she felt more comfortable, where she opened up about how hard she found medicine at times. On this day, she said, "two have gone through, two are in progress," referring to a cesarean delivery and the stillbirth patient. She explained that her role was to keep the files organized, "to see what I have to print, what is missing, for the partogram to be filled out."[5] She printed out some sheets and then cut them to the correct size required by the hospital. Half her time seemed to be spent arranging the paperwork to the hospital's specifications rather than on actual medical skills and care. Doctor Marco sat at the computer and entered patient details into the electronic medical records. Two senior residents sat on the twin bed, leaning against the wall. Doctora Valentina was sitting cross-legged, idly checking Facebook on her iPad, and Doctor Bruno, another resident, was eating his breakfast of Chocoroles (packaged jam-filled chocolate rolls) and artificial orange drink. The conversation returned to the usual concern with their work hours and their exhaustion. As Doctor Bruno munched his food, he told Doctora Valentina about a friend at another Puebla public hospital who was unhappy with his residency, commenting, "They keep them there until 9:00 P.M. [every day]." Though she chatted and checked her social media, Doctora Valentina was also in charge of the ward that morning, and she kept a keen eye on Evelyn organizing the files. After a while she asked Evelyn to check the details of "the stillbirth's" bloodwork. There was a moment's confusion, followed by laughter, as her term "óbito" (stillbirth) was heard as *"globito"* (small balloon) by Doctor Bruno. A while later the interns began sorting out paperwork for María, Carmen dictating while Paola wrote out the details: "Decrease in fetal movement. She goes to a medical center today at 9:00 [this morning]. They report fetal demise." They said that María was sent to the emergency room at Hospital Salud where the clinicians determined that there was a "lack of a heart beat [*Sin presencia de frecuencia cardiaca*]." She was later diagnosed as having hypothyroidism.[6]

Reproduction going awry (Van der Sijpt 2018) is usually best understood through a woman's or society's reproductive desires, which are deeply social (Bennett and de Kok 2018). As Sallie Han (2013) stated in her analysis of reproductive technology, the act of seeing produces the objects being seen in a different fashion from a mother's embodied experience (see also Howes-Mischel 2016; Kilshaw 2017). These fetal-imaging technologies strengthen the doctor's gaze, rendering even further the perception of mothers as vessels (Wendland 2007) and as cases rather than people. In a perverse reversal of the ways by which reproductive technology (like ultrasound) are used to reinforce the knowable reality of a live fetus in utero (Draper 2002; Han 2013; Howes-Mischel 2016; Mol 2003), in María's case the technology made the death real, knowable, measurable. In the process María's baby's social presence shifted from subject to object, and its membership in the moral community (Singer 2017) was severed. In these obstetric contexts, multiple realities of the unborn can coexist, with each constructed differently depending on where they are located, what their life status is, and who is doing the constructing (see Kilshaw 2017).

Nurse Ofelia had transferred María into the ward where other patients were in labor or held their newborns in their arms, including the cesarean patient from earlier that morning. During intake, María had said to the doctors that she could still *feel* her baby moving, but her hopes dimmed when she was told that the movement was caused by the fetus floating in the amniotic fluid and bumping against the walls of her uterus. In this terrifying transition, her baby was abruptly depersonalized, changed from a subject (my baby) to an object (the óbito, the dead fetus). She lay curled up tightly on her bed, facing the wall, her whole body seeming to silently scream her agony. Her face showed no expression, just blankness as she stared at the wall, her hand on her mouth. Her name and identity erased, she was referred to as "*la señora del óbito*"—the lady with the stillbirth— or, simply, "el óbito" by the doctors and nurses in the ward, rendering her as a case to treat rather than a suffering person.

María was given misoprostol to dilate her cervix so she could deliver her deceased baby vaginally. The medical plan was that once she was dilated, she would be given hormones to induce uterine contractions. As Erica Van der Sijpt (2018) reminds us, fetal loss is social as much as medical. Struck by the embodied horror of what the loss of a pregnancy feels like, I asked the clinicians why María did not have a cesarean surgery to remove the baby rather than allowing her to undergo the grief of going into labor with the knowledge that she would be giving birth to a dead child. "Because of the obstetric risk," was the reply from everyone: it would leave a scar, and she would have to wait to get pregnant again.

Doctora Valentina said it often took a day for the neck of the cervix to fully dilate "We wait until she can expel it (*expulsar*) in the bed." She said they would then "clamp the [cervix] and move her into the [surgery room] for a cavity revision," a painful procedure where obstetricians insert their hand into a woman's uterus to ensure that all the fetal remains and placenta are expelled from the uterus.[7] Because María's baby had died, there were different implications for the management of the loss, wherein the handling of the remains and tissue, as well as its classification (into either fetus, products of miscarriage, or stillborn child) are determined by the duration the fetus spent inside the mother (Kilshaw 2017). Doctora Valentina added that "*el producto* is very small," although the placenta was larger and would need to be delivered in a delivery room. In Mexican medical language the fetus is always impersonally referred to as el producto—the product of gestation—suggesting that only once it becomes what society intends it to be will it shift from a liminal position as an object of medical examination into a subject member of society.

How does being part of someone's life during these agonizing moments help trainee doctors learn to read the body or learn to empathize when treating patients? Do they learn about loss differently than trainees who do not face these experiences? How do these processes become embodied in the medical self? The doctors' demeanor regarding María's suffering told a deeper, more intricate story about their ideas of embodied learning, medical practice, their roles as caregivers, their individual personalities, and the ways that they connected or distanced from her. Extraordinary situations such as a stillbirth necessitate physicians learning to read everyone's emotions while also performing the "appropriate" behaviors as clinicians—stoicism, objectivity, efficacy, and competence.

Their interactions with María illuminated the duality of touch—utilitarian and practical on the one hand, and intimate and caring on the other (Van Dongen and Elema 2001). It highlighted the tension between competence in skills and caring for patients (Good 1995a). This process can be thought of as manitas on a more abstract level. As medical caregivers, clinicians become omniscient, receding emotionally from the events around them. Compassion for them is juxtaposed with their expertise. Because everyone expected her to dilate and deliver the fetus quickly, María was at first treated in a somewhat routine and dispassionate manner. Clinicians were there to do a job and attend to many patients, and so they could not take on more emotional burdens. She was touched and examined, spoken to and asked questions, but only in a detached clinical way; she was not held or physically comforted to ease her sorrow.

Obstetricians are usually not trained to deal with the emotional upheaval of a patient's grief, and they are ill equipped to provide support in these situations (Van der Sijpt 2018). The doctors often seemed to take a more pragmatic approach to these moments, telling themselves that these events were out of their hands or that they had done everything possible. At first, the interns seemed to be the only ones to feel her suffering more acutely. They had not yet learned all the ways of distancing from their patients and seemed to care more about the patients' suffering; they had not yet made the transition into medical experts. Iker thought María might develop sepsis if her baby did not emerge. He added that it must be very hard for her to be in the hospital so long, knowing that she had a dead baby in her. I agreed; I could imagine few worse things. Evelyn and Carmen said they wished they could spatially separate the patients who came in with miscarriages and stillbirths so they would not be in the same ward as the women who have their babies. As Evelyn thoughtfully put it, "One is sobbing, and the others are really happy."

It soon became evident that María's anguish and heartbreak would be prolonged. She took over thirty-six hours to slowly dilate, during which time she was kept on an intravenous drip and not allowed solid food. The doctors would periodically do tactos to determine her dilation. The day after María was admitted, she had barely dilated between one and four centimeters (there was some discrepancy in the records depending on who had done the tacto). Doctor Bruno and Doctora Valentina stood by her, gently palpating her belly. María groaned and shifted, her face furrowed in anguish, tears silently streaming down her face. They conferred among themselves and increased her dose of misoprostol, giving it to her intravenously rather than orally. Evelyn, as an intern, seemed to feel María's suffering acutely, especially the lack of solid food and familial support during this time.

Though I was familiar with the hospital policy in most Mexican public hospitals that only patients enter sterile zones—their family members and support remaining outside—I did wonder whether a situation such as María's would be a compassionate exception. However, no such exception was made, and María experienced this tragedy alone, engulfed by the activity of a bustling birthing ward. This separation further exacerbates the situation for all people involved— it brings into stark relief the clinicians' inability to emotionally support their patient, increases her isolation, and intensifies the public silence about her grief.

It is important, given how María was touched or not touched, to think about not only the context of touch in medical encounters but also the context of lack of touch. Alfonso Cuarón's Academy Award–winning film *Roma,* which was released in late 2018, has parallels to María's sorrow of losing a child in the hospital. This film narrates the story of Cleo, an Indigenous maid working for a middle-class Mexican family in early 1970s Mexico City. Cleo becomes pregnant by her boyfriend, a member of a violent paramilitary group, whose actions inadvertently cause her to go into early labor and give birth to a stillborn child. Her personal story in the film is framed by a broader critique of class, gender, and racial dynamics, of political upheaval and violence, of loss and suffering, and of health care and social structures. When we see Cleo in labor at the public hospital, it is a close-up from her side, with her body occupying the horizontal frame. All we can see of the doctors are their hands palpating her belly, doing a *tacto*, drawing out her deceased baby, and trying to resuscitate it. They appear out of focus and in shadow, while Cleo appears front and center, highlighting her personal suffering. Despite the very moving, visceral scene of loss, with the lifeless baby brought out of her body and taken by the doctors for care, none of the clinicians touch her to support her. Their touch is limited to their urgent clinical duties.[8]

There are parallels to Cleo's fictional stillbirth and María's real one. María lay in her bed alone, waiting. She was surrounded by other women in labor, other mothers. Her affect communicated her anguish and a rejection of interacting with the rest of us in the ward. Like Cleo, she was largely untouched, except for her cervix. And this touch was only to examine her dilation. No one went up to pat her, talk to her, or hug her. The omission of touch from a patient encounter—María was alone and needed comfort—is an unintended way to signal to patients and trainees that doctors are distant from those they care for, widening the gap between them. To a viewer or ethnographer, the lack of touch also suggests a significant gap in training in how to empathize with a patient's suffering.

By midmorning of María's second day in the hospital, the residents were beginning to think of possible alternatives to María's misoprostol-induced labor. They continued to undertake other duties, but María was never far from their minds. As Doctora Valentina stepped away from another surgical procedure, she said, "I hope the lady with the stillbirth does not result in a cesarean." I asked her when they would decide on this. She reiterated what they had been saying for a while: that she needed to dilate and go into labor. I once again asked why a cesarean would not be one of the options sought, to which she answered, "Because otherwise we expose her to the risks of a surgery. The *producto* is very small." Doctor Rafael, one of the most senior residents in obstetrics, said that they would only carry out a cesarean delivery on the patient "if there was any *descompensación*"—a decompensation, when primary organs begin to fail and are unable to function.

All the residents in the ward during María's stay were involved in her care, whether as direct caregivers—doing *tactos*, adjusting medications, or palpating her belly—or as indirect ones—being sounding boards for decision-making or listening to the concerns of younger trainees about her care. It was evident from people's body language and conversations that they empathized with María's prolonged suffering, and they were relieved when she finally did dilate enough for her stillborn child to emerge. (I was not there to witness it, as it occurred in the middle of her second night on the ward.) Doctor Marco later told me that hospital policy dictates that the obstetrics unit deals with a stillborn baby and not pediatrics, because it is not a live baby. They send the tiny body to the mortuary, where the family can mourn and decide what to do with their dead child (see also Susie Kilshaw's [2017] poignant elaboration of this situation in Qatar). In contrast to other contexts, by not considering María's stillborn as simply a product of gestation these social and medical practices at this hospital grant humanhood to a stillborn child, fostering the social validity of a woman's efforts to create a social and spiritual bond with her lost child (Bennett and de Kok 2018; Van der Sijpt 2018).

María's suffering allows one to understand how doctors-in-training change over time, and how they incorporate these tragedies into their medical selves. This process requires a detachment from empathy, which is most visible during these extraordinary cases. As María's suffering illustrates, she was treated at first like any other patient, even though she had an extraordinary situation. She was treated with detachment and in the ordinary ways that all patients—giving birth or giving death—were treated. But the longer she stayed in the ward and the more she suffered, her suffering became embodied and shared collectively. For two days she was a part of the ward, of people's emotions, concerns, and actions. She became central to people's fears and narratives.

Although all the doctors and trainees knew that life and death coexisted in all forms of medical care, many of them were awed by the stark juxtaposition of these forces within obstetrics wards—whereupon one baby entered life while others left it. Though many of the residents and obstetricians chose the obstetrics specialty because they enjoyed surgery, others claimed that what attracted them to the specialty was the opportunity to be part of the beginnings of someone's new life. Regardless of their reasons for being there, in their practice they moved through the ward taking care of their patients at all stages of their reproductive lives—from ordinary labor and delivery to extraordinary reproductive disruptions.

TOUCHING ONE HUNDRED PATIENTS

The doctors I met believed that one of the main ways of learning was to touch a patient—to get a feel for their bodies, for their organs, for the tissues, and how each of these could tell a story about a patient's health. In the process they gained a refined perceptual ability to discern subtle differences in the bodies of their patients (Rose 1999). Some doctors urged interns to touch as many patients as they could, to practically live and breathe the feel for a body; others believed that "sometimes one has to touch more than one hundred patients to learn something." In the process, they rendered touch explicit—refining, reinventing, and reshaping their ways of touching each time they touched and during each patient encounter (Van Dongen and Elema 2001). The interns discovered, through the repetitive actions, the intention "underlying the motion" of touching patients (Gieser 2008, 312).

Doctora Jimena Aquino was a senior physician at Hospital Piedad. She was a tall, thin woman with shoulder-length curly black hair, whose impeccably starched and ironed lab coat had its front pocket overflowing with pens. When she spoke, she enunciated every word carefully, emphasizing key words with quick hand

movements. She loved research, especially understanding the reasons for diagnoses of different cases, and claimed that she spent much time in the hospital's
archives looking at cases. This interest became especially evident during the weekly
casos clínicos. There she would ask dozens of questions in quick succession to the
interns and other doctors present.

In her office one day we spoke about her thoughts on the learning process in
medicine. Doctora Aquino began reminiscing about her own internship, years
before, at one of the most overcrowded public hospitals in the city, which had
a reputation as a fearsome training ground for medical students. Referring to
the importance of handovers for learning, she said, "We had to hand over [our
patients] to the residents. If we didn't do it, they would punish us. They [gave us]
homework, [they would] reprimand us." She added that this process "generates
learning." Like the residents who had severely scolded the Hospital Piedad
interns (which I described in chapter 3), she agreed that learning was a tactile
endeavor and could not be done in half measures. She said that the residents would
"order us to study, [tell] us to get to know the patients. We would personally do
the [patient] admission process and notify the resident: 'They have this, this, and
this.'" She added, with a proud chuckle, "We were the doctors of first contact."
Shifting her view from her own trajectory to that of the interns at Hospital Piedad, she said, "I tell them, 'Have you *felt* a uterine contraction? The uterine tone?
Is it anomalous?'⁹ They need to have the experience of [lots of] touching."

Returning to her own training, Doctora Aquino said, "The resident would tell
us, 'Go and *'pancear'* the patient." "Pancear" is a local invented verb that refers to
the *panza,* the belly (in this case of a pregnant obstetric patient), and the role of
an obstetrician in that panza; hence pancear would be the act of touching and
examining a pregnant belly, to place one's hands on the panza. Doctora Aquino
believed that these were clinical skills that all doctors-in-training must develop.
By *panceando,* trainees could tactilely develop a feel for a patient's body and its
pregnant bodily form, understanding its various dimensions, and in the process
develop their own bodies as tools for understanding those of others. She lamented
the loss of these skills among more recent trainees, blaming this loss on the reduced
opportunities for clinical contact with the patient. She added that a leading cul-
prit of this loss was clinicians' overreliance on technology, such as laboratory
tests and ultrasounds.

In her role as a senior clinician at the hospital, Doctora Aquino said she constantly reminded the interns, "Why don't you *examine* them? Why don't you
touch them?" Her words emphasize the process of enskilment (Ingold 2000), a
way of learning through doing, in a practical and material engagement with the
world—in this case, patient bodies. Doctora Aquino punctuated her argument by
concluding, "This is the inconvenience of being at a private hospital." Patients in
private hospitals have much greater bodily autonomy, and the right to determine
who can touch them and how often. Public hospital patients do not have that

privilege or right; because they depend on government funds for their health care, the patients have ceded control over much of their autonomy in these spaces. Hence, when Doctora Aquino finds private hospitals an "inconvenience," she is referring to the inability of trainees to touch, learn, and practice on as many patients as they are able.

Doctor Marco, from Hospital Salud, strongly emphasized clinical skills, particularly touch, as the central means of learning medicine: "Sometimes one has to touch more than one hundred patients to learn something." He immediately qualified this statement regarding the examination of cervical dilations through tactos, adding, "But sometimes it is not necessary to have so many patients if one has studied [the topic], if one sort of knows what [the cervix's] consistency is, and with two, three, four times one knows what a dilation is like, right? For example, in the case of dilation, it's going to be somewhat inferential, right? (*en lo de la dilatación siempre va a ser algo muy sugestivo, ¿no?*). Why? Because our hands are our tools." That is, tactos are not a precise or standard system of measurement, and they are performed by empirically sensing and applying one's cultural meaning to the "sensory substrate" (Csordas 1993, 148). The process is about somatically translating a nonstandard system into a more standard one, while still acknowledging some of its lack of precision. We saw this inferential nature of *tacto* measurements in the disagreement over how dilated María was during her stay in the ward for her stillbirth.

Despite spending many hours in the delivery wards at both hospitals over the years of this research, I witnessed only *one* vaginal birth. In a sad and strange paradox, it is important to remember that María was made to deliver her stillborn child vaginally, while cesareans and other surgical medical interventions seemed to be reserved for the living. The one "true" vaginal birth experience I saw was the birth of Graciela's second child. Graciela underwent labor on one of the gurneys in the ward of Hospital Salud. She was connected to an intravenous bag of fluids and Pitocin, and she was supported by some of the staff (I have a longer description of this birth in Dixon, Smith-Oka, and El Kotni 2019). Graciela did not receive an epidural because, as I mentioned before, pain relief is a scarce resource.

One of the attending obstetricians at the hospital, Doctor Tadeo Molina, exemplified the attitude of using touch as a means to expedite obstetric procedures.[10] Because vaginal births were so rare, on this day Graciela was the focus of all the clinicians' attention. (At one point I counted fourteen clinicians surrounding her, which included several interns as well as first-year residents on their first day of residency.) Doctor Molina was a tall man in his mid-thirties, with a small beard and a heavy brow; his good looks accentuated his cockiness. The hospital hierarchy was strictly enforced: Doctora Valentina, the senior resident, had been in charge of the ward when they were caring for María; but the moment an attending physician, especially a male physician, took over care, Doctora Valentina's status reverted to that of a junior and trainee.

Today Doctor Molina focused on training his residents to accelerate cervical dilation through tactos and manual dilation, an obstetrically violent form of practice that I have described in previous work as a bureaucratic and routine practice (Smith-Oka 2013a). Putting his hand into Graciela's vagina, causing her to cry out, he said in a matter-of-fact voice, "Her pelvis is small. I have just broken her membranes." As he pulled off his glove, he said, "Now the [amniotic] sac is broken, the baby will engage (*encajar*). Let's give it a chance." He then turned to Doctora Valentina and told her that, as an obstetrician/gynecologist, she should properly "learn what labor is like, as it is our daily bread." Daily bread, as a Christian religious symbol of God's love, likens the labor of doctors to divine caregivers. Devotees are meant to humbly speak the Lord's Prayer to ask for basic food to sustain their life day to day. This doctor's words suggest that their medical labor was humble and ordinary, sharply contrasting with how he encouraged his trainees to act in Graciela's care—with arrogance and violence.

Doctor Molina instructed Doctora Valentina: "When you feel it, you dilate them manually." He demonstrated to her and Doctor Marco how to dilate a cervix by again putting his fingers into Graciela, palm facing up. His gloves were covered in blood and tissue as he showed his residents how to do this maneuver. Evelyn and Paola, the two interns that day, stood to the side, observing these procedures. Pulling out his glove from Graciela's vagina, Doctor Molina turned to Doctor Marco, ordering him, "Touch her." Doctor Marco put on a glove and inserted his own hand, telling Graciela, "A small discomfort, I'm just going to see." He was gentler and humbler than Doctor Molina, his arrogance not yet cemented. Doctor Molina stood by Doctor Marco, saying, "She is more effaced." He demonstrated on his own hands how to efface the cervix so the baby's head could descend. He told his residents that this was the main maneuver they needed to know and do, saying, "You'll see that once we take these [membranes] away how quickly [the baby] comes out." He bragged that as a senior resident at another public hospital he would do a whole series of these dilations in a row, making his junior residents panic with the increased number of patients in active labor.

When does the human body become an instrument of learning? On this day Doctor Molina used Graciela as a teaching tool—inserting his hands or asking one of his residents to insert theirs—to teach the trainees how to do the maneuver as well as to accelerate Graciela's contractions. Ignoring her cries of pain, he crowed, "How long did we take to dilate her? Not everyone knows how to do this. We saved her three hours of labor." In doing so, the treatment toward Graciela was obstetrically violent, where her wishes and needs were not consulted, her body was completely exposed to the view of multiple clinicians, and she never consented to the uncomfortable and painful procedures to which she was subjected. Doctor Molina's focus on the temporal pace of labor grotesquely depersonalized Graciela, and she simply became an object for practice and demonstration.

Doctor Molina soon gave the order for Graciela to be rolled into the delivery room. Although she seemed relieved to be moved into delivery, she had had no decision-making power at any point during the labor and delivery. The younger residents and interns placed her legs in stirrups. She was screaming in pain. A female resident cleaned Graciela's legs and vaginal area with antiseptic. It was decided that Doctor Marco would attend. He began by cutting an episiotomy, a routine procedure for this hospital and most others across the country where a woman's perineum is cut to widen the vaginal opening for delivery. Doctor Molina pressed on Graciela's abdomen.[11] As the baby's head crowned, every clinician looked on expectantly. Graciela's baby girl was born at 12:17 P.M. Doctor Marco held the baby as another resident helped him to cut the cord. Graciela sighed, "My baby is out." The pediatrician holding the baby placed her gently on Graciela's chest. Graciela gasped in delight. The baby was then taken by the pediatrics team to clean and measure.

An overarching theme woven through the cases I describe in this chapter is how the bodies of medical practitioners can traverse boundaries, whether in cutting during a cesarean delivery, doing a tacto on a laboring or stillbirth patient, or manually dilating a cervix to expedite birth. It is also about how patients are seen or unseen as objects of care, teaching, or practice. Byron Good (1994) stated that *seeing* the body is invasive because it crosses boundaries. However, unseeing a patient can be equally violent: depersonalizing, utterly medicalizing, and reducing them to cases or objects under observation. The medical hand can cross boundaries that other hands cannot. Doctors can touch patients by following social scripts (Henslin and Biggs 1971; Teman 2010) in ways and in places that would not be allowed in other contexts or by other people.

Medical hands can cross socially scripted boundaries of intimacy; social scripts make the actions of medical hands (touching people's bodies) seem "normal" and ordinary, which in other situations would be socially unacceptable. Only in medical contexts, such as the ones I have described, can the intimate type of touching take place without there being any intimacy at all. Reversing ordinary and extraordinary structures, the medical hand can enter into a person's body, and doctors' eyes can see parts of the body that are usually reserved for personal or intimate spaces. Conversely, when intimate and caring touch is needed, as for a grieving patient, that touch is usually absent. Medical practices can cross these boundaries because of the social script that convenes the roles that doctors and patients can play—how patients cede control and privacy over their body, and how doctors touch, probe, prod, cut, or even hurt within this given context and this given script.

Ultimately, by crossing these boundaries, trainees embody their emerging authority as physicians in training. Trainees cultivated assertiveness and competence over the course of their interactions with patients, learning when to empathize with and when to detach from patient suffering, and mastering their expertise in using their bodies as tools within medical spaces. During the process of acquiring a medical self, trainees engage in structural exercises where they mimic and enact the expected dispositions of medicine, and they learn about the ability and the perceived right to manipulate the body of a patient, which is paramount to the care and their role as physicians.

Trainees move from the periphery of the medical action—managing instruments and paperwork—to the center of the action as they shift from trainees to experts. This shift is evident in the ways that interns describe their enskilment—as Lupe did in narrating her gradual transition from blindness into sightedness—and the increased responsibility for patient care interns have by the end of their internship. In their final days as interns, they emphasized their increased competence in skills and their greater ease with hospital practices, learning, "clinical reasoning, patient examinations, note write-up, and arriving at diagnoses . . . and knowing what treatments to give patients, because now I will be the one in charge of them." Others focused on the interpersonal as a means to obtain patient compliance: "I think the most important [skill] is to learn to relate well to the patient, because when they trust you it's easier to get them to see their disease and for them to follow the treatment." These bodily practices ultimately reinforce their position of authority within the patient encounter.

CONCLUSION
Medicine as an Imperfect System

Medicine is an art. It's not an exact science. There are people who study music, and by reading the sheet music they can interpret a great song; in the same way there are people who without the sheet music can play that same melody with the same passion and the same feeling.
>—Doctor Jesús Morales, physician at Hospital Piedad

The internship should not be rose-tinted; *se les consiente demasiado* [you are too pampered].
>——Doctor Bernardo Villalpando, physician at Hospital Piedad

I think that is one of the things that has made the most change on me: you witness the suffering and pain of the people and you say, "I have to do my job even better."
>—Amanda, intern at Hospital Piedad

The research for this book began with a journey. It was a long journey, and a personal one. It began with my work almost two decades ago in a Mexican Indigenous village where the women I met described feeling pressured by doctors and nurses to conform to a particular way of mothering that oftentimes contradicted their own cultural ways. My journey then took me to the city of Puebla, where I found myself doing ethnography in a very busy public hospital where I witnessed the mistreatment of women who did not fit with perceptions of good mothers—the women who were unmarried, who were adolescent, or who were poor or Indigenous. I held women as they cried in pain, fear, or loneliness, and I could not answer their questions of why the doctors treated them that way. Like many scholars before me, my writings criticized the doctors for their actions and for their violence.

I began the third leg of my journey to understand why. Why were these doctors treating their patients this way? Were they inherently violent? Did I just happen to be researching a rogue hospital or ward? Was the aggression learned in

medical school? Was it more deeply woven into society? What I found were par-
tial answers. And they were humbling. Some doctors were rogue—they appeared
distant or callous, seeming to not care much for who their patients were or what
they felt. Some of them proudly transmitted these practices and beliefs to their
juniors, perpetuating the violence in those wards. Some hospitals and wards were
known for more aggressive forms of treatment because of their doctors' exhaustion, impatience, or inability to find the time to care for everyone. But most doctors were not inherently violent; they were simply trying to do their best under
sometimes hard circumstances where, though empathy was one of their "primary moral resources" (Luhrmann 2000, 280), it was sometimes in short supply.
The broader political economy of care significantly shaped how doctors practiced. They worked with the available supplies and infrastructure; they worked
despite long shifts that demanded that their human bodies behave like machines;
they worked at reconciling the overt and hidden parts of the curriculum; and they
worked at caring for patients even within an internally and externally violent
system.

This book is also a journey of interns transforming their medical self. Medical
selving is a process shaped by specific contexts and circumstances, and influenced by the efforts and will of each trainee. It is a deep and mindful reshaping of
the body and mind. Medical selving begins with the outward appearance—the
clothes and emblems that convey doctorly affects to others. But trainees gradually incorporate self-making changes that go deep into the self, which becomes a
new way of knowing and being. Medical selves are acquired, embodied, and also
performed.

The embodied nature of the medical self and the process of medical selving
are what distinguish this from other processes of identity formation. The medical
self is nuanced, flexible, and fluid; it is shaped both by the broader history and
political economy of medicine and by the particular ways of doing things in different spaces. No two people's medical self is ever the same. The interns at Hospital Salud who attended to María's stillbirth would have developed a different
understanding of loss than the interns at Hospital Piedad who attended the code
red. The female interns who were harassed would have emerged from their medical training with a different understanding of gender relations within the medical profession than their male peers who experienced *mano dura*. The interns at
both hospitals who persisted in attending surgeries as *instrumentistas* and first
assistants would have a different perspective on surgical tools than others. Those
who made large mistakes would emerge from the internship with a different
appreciation for practice and safety than those who did not experience these.

In many of the interactions I have described in this book we can see how the
broader gendered, racialized, and classed structures of Mexico are reproduced
through the training of medical students. Despite being contextually and individually specific, medical selving is also a universal process for medical trainees

anywhere. The surgeons in Rachel Prentice's (2013) work in the United States incorporated grueling ethical, technical, and emotional skills in order to learn how to cut into the bodies of patients, while doing so against a backdrop of increased technological practice. In Beatriz Reyes-Foster's (2018) ethnography, the psychiatrists in Mexico had to negotiate meanings of truth and madness in encounters with their patients, while those in Tanya Luhrmann's (2000) haunting work in the United States were concerned with their moral responsibility. The Malawian medical students described by Claire Wendland (2010) learned to be creative and resourceful within a profoundly resource-poor setting.

What I illustrate in this book is that medicine is an imperfect system. Though doctors are an extension of God's hand, they are not gods themselves because doctors are fallible and flawed. Whether doing art or science, most doctors are simply trying to do their best. Simultaneously, most patients are just hoping to get out of the hospital unharmed. As the opening quote from Doctor Morales states, doctors must have passion and feeling to truly "play the melody" of medicine. Seeming to eschew the connection between medicine as science and medicine's prestige, he added that he was not implying that people didn't have to learn medicine but that "to have that ability to recognize a patient's illness, one does need a gift. Experience can substitute for the gift. There are very experienced doctors who already have that skill to diagnose—and that's bestowed through many years of practice. And there are people who are born with that ability to easily recognize illness." In his words he suggests a gift beyond prosaic bodily skill that is only bestowed on certain people, making them extraordinary doctors. But he also suggests that medical providers can become gifted at healing through deliberate and lengthy practice in developing their abilities and skills.

With this book, I contribute to a growing conversation in anthropology about how social structures perpetuate themselves. The transformational processes of medical selving guide people's behaviors unconsciously through their bodily and sensorial ways of being as well as through broader institutional forces that shape who they are. But medical selves are also consciously produced and deliberately cultivated, where trainees decide what kind of a medical self they aim to create in their journeys through medicine. Medical selving is a total transformation.

In institutions such as hospitals, the ordinary and the extraordinary are two sides of the same coin, blending to the point of indistinctiveness, where bodies occupy space in certain ways and must navigate it through somatic means. Ordinary medical practice is where medical selving is most profound, as trainees repeat and practice skills until they gain mastery, like interns did as instrumentistas, for instance. But the heightened emotions and sensorial awareness produced during extraordinary moments—patients suffering, unexpected events—created the important substrate for the solidification of their medical selves. The approach I have used in the book can help to explain how assumptions, values, knowledge, practices, and skills are transmitted to the next generations for the ultimate purpose of maintaining institutions' effectiveness through time. It explains the logics of medicine, and how they unfold within spaces and between people.

I have provided a close-up of the lives of doctors and trainees backstage, and through this I allow readers entry into spaces not usually accessible to the public. What I show is that the medical self is a whole new way of seeing and sensing and is constantly being shaped and attuned through the use of medical artifacts, new approaches to practice, narratives to "en-case" patients (Holmes and Ponte 2011), mistakes that reconceptualize knowledge, and the invisible assumptions that structure ideals about good medicine and good doctoring. Medical students enter the internship composed of an existing sense of self, which has been formed over their lived experiences as individuals as well as mutually articulated and in an "embodied presence" (Csordas 1993, 138) with people around them. Medical selving is about the boundary between self and others while also collapsing distinctions between subject and object, which allows an investigation into how cultural objects (including selves) are constituted or objectified (Csordas 1990, 39).

Though medical trainees are subjects, in their journey through medical school they can sometimes become objects of training, a process that simultaneously connects them to other medical people and separates them from those who are not medical. I highlight the ambiguous position interns have within the medical hierarchy: as interns they are no longer medical students, but they are also not yet doctors. I have, in describing this, helped readers understand how doctors-in-training change over time, and how they somatically transform into their expert persona, learning to read the patient's body with their own, making them both legible. Interns are in the process of becoming experts. They are able to wield medical technology, skills, and language with greater ease, and this ease becomes more apparent by the end of their internship as they gain more expertise with tools, seeing them as extensions of the self.

Throughout training, the trainees' authority and abilities are questioned by the "real" experts. The oft-repeated adage to interns was that they had to ignore their pride and ask for help: "Always ask, 'hey, I don't know, tell me,' [because] knowledge is fundamental." Doctor Navarro reminded interns that not only should they ask, gain knowledge, and act according to norms and policies, but they also must understand the role of resources in medical care. He said, "The better the resources [and] instruments, so will the quality of care be better." He described what he considered to be the four essential elements for good care: "One, prevent the damage—that is, improve health. Another, attend to the damage—that is, medical attention. But there are two fundamental ones: research and teaching. Research is not investigating to discover something new; it's investigating to discover what's already there, what's evident, the essential." Returning full circle to the need to ask questions as part of teaching and learning, Doctor Navarro described how he and Doctor García had recently attended to a woman who had been in a bad accident:

We hospitalized her, and the lady was anxious because her [three-month-old baby] was at home unable to breastfeed and the mother had her breasts [full of milk] and was in tremendous pain. But the clinical history never said that the woman had given birth. Why does that matter? Because of the type of analgesic prescribed. [He reiterated that interns must ask] twenty-one times why. . . . "Why are you overweight?" "Ah, because I eat a lot." "Why do you eat a lot?" "Because I have little time." "Why do you have little time?" "Because I am disorganized in my activities." "Why don't you become more organized?" "Because I need money." So the whys [allow one] to find the root of the problem, and a solution can be given.

Doctor Navarro's words emphasize the main underpinnings of medical selving. It is about enskilment: simultaneously learning and doing, asking and probing, knowing and caring. It melds self with the objects of medicine—the tools, the techniques, the language—embodying them during practice. It is about losing one's fear of crossing intimacy boundaries and learning to cut, pierce, or touch. These are all gained through practice and taking what is already known about medicine to diagnose and treat a patient. Although practice is repetitive, it is not mindless. It is a bodily and mindful endeavor, incorporating all the values, skills, attitudes, practices of medicine into the medical self.

By being a part of a patient's life during moments of joy or heartache, interns learn to train their bodies—hands, eyes, ears—to see (and unsee) the bodies of their patients. Within medical selving is the creation, crossing, and blurring of boundaries. These processes form a central part of the logics of medicine. These are boundaries between bodies, between flesh and technology, between which patients can be practiced upon and which not, between victims and perpetrators of gender-based violence, and between the performances that occur frontstage and those that take place backstage. Doctors' hands could cross the bodily and social boundaries of their patients; interns' bodies gradually shift from novices to experts with each new practice and skill, shedding some of their fears and apprehensions as they gain confidence.

As the trainees moved up the hierarchy, they were permitted to cross even more boundaries; as they became more expert, they moved from the periphery to the center of medical practice. They started by only being able to cross minor boundaries of the skin through sutures and blood draws, progressed to being able to perform tactos; and eventually were allowed to cut into a woman's body during a cesarean delivery. The rules by which they were first bound dissolved; with each new skill, the boundary between them and their patients thinned. Their patients' bodies became contingently more permeable, and the boundary between doctor and patient blurred, becoming a contested place of practice.

By learning to wield instruments and by using their patients' bodies as instruments of learning, the trainees blurred boundaries between flesh and technology. They became increasingly cyborg as their bodies incorporated technological implements—scalpels to enter into the bodies of others, ultrasounds and Doppler scans to see and hear the body's insides, and even cellphones to keep track of all patients under the hospital's care. By incorporating technology as a replacement for direct human interaction, they were also learning to unsee. They learned to view people as patients, and patients as cases, in what Prentice called an ontological duality (2013, 257), where a person can also be an object; but remnants of patients' personhood can also bring the case/patient's "personhood into view."

The process of unseeing was evident in the boundary between public and private patients, evincing Khiara Bridges' (2011) racial, but also classed and gendered, geography. Everyone knew that public patients were available for practice and there were fewer boundaries between practitioner and patient, but few people seemed to try to change the system. They saw the reality but were (sometimes) blind to its effects. They often learned to unsee the priorities of their patients, instead prioritizing their own clinical temporalities (Andaya 2019). As Janelle Taylor and Claire Wendland have stated, "Institutions of education systematically teach people to *unsee* their social world in ways that contribute to the maintenance of existing social relations of class and power—but education *could* teach people to *see* their world clearly, and support their capacity to transform it" (2015, 57, emphasis in original).

When Hospital Piedad was under recertification, the entire staff intently prepared over the course of several weeks. The interns were given strict orders to portray professionalism, wear their complete and tidy uniform, and memorize their intern manual in case they were quizzed by the assessors. They were placed on shorter shifts so they would not encounter the assessors too often and so there would not be questions about the ratio of twenty-two interns to forty hospital beds. Many of these requests were for performative purposes so the hospital directors could show the assessors how well they functioned as a teaching hospital. However, during these weeks some doctors also focused on teaching their trainees to think more deeply about their patients' social circumstances.

At one meeting Doctora Aquino told the interns to think about patients' situation before sending them home, "Because if you tell them, 'You have to eat twenty grams of cottage cheese,' and the patient lives in the [*sierra*], well, how nice, but there's not going to be any cottage cheese there." Another doctor added that they needed to think about what they would do if they sent insulin home with a patient who "didn't have anywhere at home to keep it cold." Doctora Aquino suggested a "tropicalized alternative": taking in the patient's environment so there would be better adherence to the treatment and hence reduce risk. She said this was "part of the hospital recertification standards, which is called 'education for the patient and their family.' If we don't educate them well, they will commit medication errors that could even cost them their life." She added that doctors needed to send patients home with specific instructions: "If they have an appointment in four weeks; if the medication is for three days; if the diet is forever. So, all that might seem silly, but the patient does not have medical common sense, they don't know what we're thinking when we are discharging them." She concluded, "So, I think that we do have to take all that into account: the patient's psychosocial environment so we can achieve a better adherence to the [medical] recommendations."

What this story and many others in the book illustrate is the complexity and nuance within medical training and hospital care. Trainees did not simply learn about medical practice; they learned to incorporate the principles and values of these medical institutions into their daily practice. They learned these through overt teaching by mentors as well as through the hidden curriculum, which taught the interns how things worked there, what was valued, why they needed to care, and what was "medical common sense." Doctors can be skilled at performing a detailed medical examination and history taking, but the temporal realities of care mean that they sometimes have to use their available time to distill the "important" parts of the patient into the clinical case. Sometimes they do have time to ask all the questions suggested by Doctor Navarro and to pay attention to a patient's psychosocial environment, but other times they do not. This can create a disjoint between telling a patient's story and editing out details that might not feel important. There was violence within some of the care, with situations that evinced the perceived value and worth of different populations. These practices underscored the hierarchy of prestige present in hospital spaces—about who belonged and how, whose practice had more value and why.

Despite medical training being ostensibly objective, many of the stories in this book are illustrative of how deep structural perceptions about gender, class, race, or color were subjectively reproduced, acquired, and perpetuated in medical training. Some physicians tried to pay close attention to these structures and worked to improve them, like Amanda's words at the start of the chapter, where she deliberately focused on alleviating her patients' pain and suffering or Doctora Aquino's suggestion to tropicalize their medical care. There were many examples of dignity toward patients and of doctors exhorting interns to care about their vulnerable patients, like Doctor Contreras's urging doctors to reflect their own life upon ways of being a doctor. Though there was bullying and abuse of authority as well as concerns with external violence on the medical profession, some people managed to address these, protest these, or, at the very least, laugh about these with others.

Because of the structures internal to hospitals, women doctors occupied a different space than their male counterparts. Women worked hard to show that they belonged. However, their male peers also had to learn to manage the effect of harsher mano dura during their training, especially when interacting with more toxically masculine senior physicians. Female doctors experienced duality in these spaces: they not only were expected to learn the skills and techniques like any other medical student, but they also endured problematic gender harassment, transactional bargaining, power dynamics, or gender-based violence in order to thrive (or survive). But the boundary between them as victims and as perpetrators was also evident, and sometimes blurred. Their intersectionality was evident in their interactions with male peers and with female patients. In the former their gender made them inferior; in the latter their social and economic capital within Mexico's pigmentocracy made them superior.

Ultimately, the issues I raise about medical training and practice, and the reproduction of structural violence within and outside of the walls of medicine, are not a story unique to Mexico, or even limited to low-resource hospitals and settings. As Gabriela Soto Laveaga and Claudia Agostoni (2011) have argued, the health system in Mexico has increasingly pitted patients and health-care providers against each other. Doctors reinforce their value-laden perceptions during their encounters with patients. Each group sees the other as the aggressor—patients are seen to be gaming the system, using it too much, not listening to doctors' expert advice, and making the lives of doctors harder; doctors are seen to be providing questionable care or withholding it altogether. More seasoned doctors knew that the year of social service truly pitted both groups against each other.

When violence toward patients did occur—and, as I have shown in this book, it did happen, sometimes frequently—it tended to be situational violence. That is, it was a reflection of problematic structures, where two-dimensional timetables and protocols were enacted on three-dimensional, living patients or where overworked doctors at public hospitals hurried patients through the system by "treating them like cows," as Julieta described it. Though trainees were encouraged to pay attention to their patients' social and economic background, many times these circumstances were dismissed as *cultura* or beliefs that needed to be moved past in order to provide care. Some of these perceptions about patients emerged from historically discriminatory, stratified moral regimes of "cultural" hierarchies and values, where some populations were seen to lack the necessary cultural practices for being good patients and good citizens, or where purchasing power translated into better caregiving.

Since my original research, there have been a few changes to the medical training system. The change most significant to medical trainees was to the *guardias*. In 2018 the Mexican government officially established that interns and residents should have no more than two overnight shifts per week rather than three, so they had three days to rest between each guardia. The length of each guardia remains the same at thirty-two hours. Some of the former interns, who missed this change by a couple of years, agreed that it was an important change but that the structure continued to signal to trainees that their labor was needed solely to fill the gaps in hospital care and to "shape [trainees'] medical character." Another important change was the prohibition of *guardias de castigo*—the punishment shifts where trainees could be forced by others senior to them to stay beyond their work hours in the hospital. These do not appear to have disappeared completely, and the deeper violence within the hierarchical interactions remains.

The labor of doctors working in medical spaces is not always easy, and, as the stories throughout the book illustrate, it took endurance and creativity to continue practicing medicine despite the difficulties. Given Mexico's rocky history with health, it is unlikely that these difficulties will disappear. The new health system changes are designed with universal health care in mind to provide care to populations without insurance. Anyone with a national identification card can now go to any public hospital—Mexican Institute for Social Security [IMSS], Security and Social Services for Workers of the State [ISSSTE], or Ministry of Health—and be attended for free (Instituto de Salud para el Bienestar [INSABI] 2020), though there has been significant concern that Mexico is not investing enough in health care and infrastructure to achieve this goal (Mendoza Escamilla 2019). Although the plan was to increase the number of clinicians through additional incentives, this change was not yet visible by the writing of this book. People were very concerned about even more overcrowding in the already overcrowded system. And although part of the new health budget was allotted to increase the number of jobs, many of these will be in remote, underserved places. As Kevin explained, although the plan is laudable and will potentially bring biomedical care to populations that need it, few doctors want to work in isolated sierra communities. In those places, he claimed, there is still a lack of appropriate infrastructure, instruments, supplies, and even a lack of food in some of the communities, where doctors must rely on the generosity of the population for meals or water. As he asked, despite the higher salaries, who wants to work in such extreme circumstances?

Paola said, when we spoke on the phone a few years after she had completed her internship, that Mexico "always needs doctors." Large pharmacy chains across the nation are capitalizing on the surfeit of young general practitioners who need jobs, and most have added consultation rooms to their pharmacies. One study calculates that approximately 41 percent of private ambulatory medical consultations take place at these pharmacies (Díaz-Portillo et al. 2015). The marketization of medical skills, where patients can comparison shop for the least expensive care option (even as low as 25 pesos, which is just over U.S.$1), puts enormous pressure on these doctors to be competitive and cut their rates, which my interlocutors saw as a process of doctors "selling their labor" at "lower prices than even hairstylists." The gap in health care is being filled by those most vulnerable in the system—in this case, by the underpaid young general practitioners. Although this topic is beyond the scope of this book, questions of precarity, deprofessionalization, and even deskilling are important and relatively understudied phenomena, and they merit closer anthropological attention.

I have kept in touch with many of the participants. Some chose not to take the national residency examination and work as general practitioners, either in private practice, public hospitals, or in pharmacies. Each year approximately 50,000 applicants take the residency examination, of which fewer than 10 percent pass. Even after passing, the chances of finding a residency position are not easy; some hospitals receive hundreds of applicants and accept only a handful of residencies. Despite these hurdles, some of my interlocutors are now in their residency (or about to enter it)—whether in Puebla, other regions of Mexico, or abroad. Some passed their residency exams on their first try and entered the residency of their choice. Others took time to work or study in order to pass their exams—some are still waiting to do that. Some have enrolled in additional degree programs—such as for a masters in administration of medical institutions—that could provide them with additional opportunities for employment later in their careers. They all seemed to be happy with their lives and their choice to be doctors.

"What's important now is not what happened, but what *will* happen. What is your future? Where will you all work within five, seven, ten years?" said Doctor Navarro to the interns at one of the last *casos clínicos* I attended, where Samantha was the presenter. The doctors at the event spoke about the changes they had seen over the years and those that they could expect in the future. Doctor Navarro told the interns that "the future of hospitals are the acute [cases]. . . . What is most expensive in medical care is hospitalization; the hospital gets the most dough from this." He added that even private hospitals like Hospital Piedad have limitations, but he saw these changes as a good challenge within "a business like ours" to apply good technology to treat patients in a less expensive manner. Focusing on the significant ways that the economics of health care structure patient access, he said that hospitals could not run without money: "*Con dinero baila el perro* [Money will make the dog dance], . . . and now our [financial] director says, 'Without money there's no admission.'" He continued, trying to find a solution to these financial constraints in care; "And so, obviously, we have to reduce the hospitalization times. From here come the minimally invasive or ambulatory surgeries. . . . And obviously, like always, to manage pain; no one has the right to feel pain." He explained what acute care meant for the hospital and for training: "This [hospital] will attend precisely to the acute ills, the accidents, which you know we have many, or the aggravation of chronic cases. This [change] definitely improves surgical techniques." Returning to the need to practice and develop competence, he told the interns that "if you don't know, don't go in [to a procedure]." He concluded, with a laugh, "The most dangerous thing in a hospital is a doctor with initiative and no knowledge."

The ambiguity of interns within the system and their concomitant fear of leaving the relative safety of the internship were dramatically heightened the closer they got to the end of their internship and the beginning of their mandatory year of social service. For their mandatory year the trainees would be sent to underserved places—usually on their own—to be entirely responsible for the care of patients for the very first time. Some of the interns were excited about this next phase: they would have the ability to wield their moral and symbolic power in their practice of medicine (Soto Laveaga 2013b) and contribute to improving the health and lives of impoverished people across the country. But most expressed fears about their abilities and expertise in real-life cases far from their hospital base, and they wondered if they had enough needed skills and knowledge—they did not want to be that "most dangerous thing" that Doctor Navarro described. They were also very fearful of the potential to be affected by the endemic violence of which doctors had increasingly become victims. The women were especially vocal in their fears about sexual violence and femicides; years later, some of the women shared that because they were the only doctor at their post, they would lock themselves into their room at the clinic every night for fear of being victims of violence.

Doctor Santiago, the anesthesiology resident at Hospital Salud, worried about the welfare of underprepared interns, and he phrased his concerns as a Self–Other between clinicians and patients: "They're going to be alone. . . . People in some of the [rural] communities are very aggressive. And if a doctor lets a baby die due to negligence, they will kill him for that." Echoing what Doctor Navarro said previously, Doctor Santiago would tell the interns, "In your life something will happen one day, but you should be able to say, 'The patient's [condition] got complicated because I didn't have the supplies, because I didn't have some [necessity], whatever.' But you should never be able to say, 'I complicated [their condition] because of having acted incorrectly, because I didn't know, or because of negligence.'"

When we last spoke in early 2020, Kevin was about to begin his residency in Mexico City. He recounted how he had experienced several chilling moments of violence during his year of social service, where he had attended to hurt members of armed gasoline theft rings (called *huachicoleros*) and was threatened with physical violence amid "a parade of guns" in the clinic. Perhaps due to a combination of his tall stature and calm character and the vital medical role he played in the community, he remained unharmed and even managed to establish a détente-like rapport with the local gang leader. Despite this experience, Kevin's optimism remained. The year of social service had cemented his vocation for medicine and his aim to contribute to the improvement of people's health.

When we spoke a couple of years after the end of his internship at Hospital Piedad, Gabriel said he saw his role as that of a ship's captain: working toward keeping the sinking system afloat. He chose to do part of his training abroad, but his plan was to return to Mexico afterward to contribute toward the betterment of its health care. Like many of his peers, he had criticized the medical system in Mexico. But he also described how his year of social service at a mobile clinic had provided medical care to a large catchment area of impoverished rural communities. He had seen the positive effects the national health programs had on improving people's access to medicine and reducing mortality and morbidity. The clinical spaces and their doctors were the means for patients to "at least have basic contact with a doctor." He worried about the rapidly changing health-care structure and its effects on doctors and patients, especially the sharp cuts in health-care budgets, which directly affected supplies, medications, clinicians' jobs and salaries, and other necessities for providing care.

I finished revisions to this book in mid-2020, during the novel coronavirus pandemic. The doctors of my acquaintance were struggling to comprehend the magnitude of this issue within a medical system already strained under normal circumstances. Both news sources and my medical friends emphasized the fear among medical providers at both public and private hospitals: fear of becoming victims of COVID-19 but also fear of becoming victims of violence that can "cause the deaths of more physicians" (Briseño 2020). Calculations in August 2020 suggested that over one-fifth of COVID-19 infections in Mexico were of medical personnel (one of the highest rates in the world) and that over 1,000 workers had already died of the disease (Reuters 2020). By the end of 2020, Mexico had the highest death rate worldwide of medical workers due to COVID-19 (Amnistía Internacional 2020). Several hospitals lost much of their staff due to illness or absenteeism (Kitroeff and Villegas 2020).

We must stop to think: If, under "normal" circumstances the medical system is strained, how can it—and its workers—survive a situation such as COVID-19? What sorts of effects will this situation have on the immediate and long-term health and well-being of health-care providers? How can these doctors and nurses provide medical care to patients under increasingly strained systems? If medical selving is a total transformation, whereby fledgling doctors are trained to change their affect, bodily engagement, language, views on the world, and ways of thinking, how do extremely transformative situations such as pandemics impact their selves? What do providers learn from these situations, and how do they incorporate them into their medical selves?

Many doctors might need to recall skills learned when they were trainees or learn new techniques in their efforts to attend to patients with a novel disease, serving as a reminder to them that their medical self is never quite fixed. Others might need to overcome their fear in order to continue their work (Camacho Servín 2020). Situations such as this show that the process of medical selving continues long after medical trainees become fledgling residents and god-like attending physicians. While some practices, values, and attitudes are cemented along the way, most doctors keep learning and molding their minds and bodies to continue inhabiting their medical selves—both consciously and unconsciously—in their professional journey. The malleability of the medical self means that it grows with doctors as they undergo their "doctorly" experiences, whether under normal, unexpected, or catastrophic conditions. Their medical transformation is lengthy, painful, and gut wrenching as they strive to reduce the suffering of their patients. But its totality means that they are never *not* doctors: their medical self is a permanent part of their selves.

The interns I met were unique as individuals, but they were similar to interns across Mexico. They had a combination of drives and concerns for providing care; some had a greater commitment than others to "accept responsibility for the health of a patient," which Doctor Morales considered to be the basic principle for doctors. As Samantha wistfully said, "I would really like all people to receive the same type of medical care." Given what I know about them and how they think about their role within larger Mexico, I hope that they will be able to achieve their dreams of transforming medical care in Mexico, foster an environment where both doctors and patients are treated with dignity, pay more attention to the violence within the system, and aim to change the way medicine is taught and practiced.

ACKNOWLEDGMENTS

I owe the existence of this book to very many people. First and foremost are the interns who allowed me entry into their medical lives. Though I have shared their lives in the pages of this book pseudonymously, I hope I have done justice to their dreams, lives, joys, and travails. I have been fortunate to make their friendships. They generously gave of their time to answer my questions, inviting me into procedures, classes, and handovers, and also welcoming me into their own spaces of familiarity—their residences, downtimes, and meals, and even letting Megan and I use one of their beds, depriving some of them of a better night's sleep. I know I was sometimes in their way and my questions were not always sage or wise, and yet they never gave up on me. When the book was almost done and I let them all know, they responded with excitement and eagerness to talk about where they were and what they were doing, taking time away from their work as residents and doctors to talk with me. I owe them an infinite debt of thanks. This book is for all of them. Though I cannot name them individually, the residents, attending doctors, and directors at the hospitals were generous, kind, and welcoming of my research. I am thankful for their trust in allowing me access to these hospital spaces and in permitting me to be a small part of their lives. They were generous in answering questions, in teaching me how to walk and talk like a doctor, and in showing me the complexities of medical life.

The research for this book was funded by various sources over the years, such as the Helen Kellogg Institute for International Studies, the Institute for Scholarship in the Liberal Arts, and the Eck Institute for Global Health, all at the University of Notre Dame. Several people at these institutes were instrumental in supporting this intellectual endeavor, particularly Sharon Schierling, Paolo Carrozzo, Steve Reifenberg, Lori Loftis, Anne Hayes, Katherine Taylor, Bernard Nahlen, and Tom Merluzzi.

Key people in Puebla supported this project with infrastructure, advice, transport, and even food. Lisette Monterroso has been supportive and welcoming from the very start of my work in Puebla so very long ago: finding me lodging, feeding me, introducing me to the beauties of the city, and even helping to find a lovely kindergarten for my daughter. I could not have done this work without her friendship. I lived in Olivia del Bosque's guesthouse for much of this work, and her care toward me, my students, and my daughter were unparalleled. When I met Elena Soto-Vega at the medical school at the Universidad Popular Autónoma del Estado de Puebla (UPAEP), I knew I had found a kindred spirit. Over the years, and lots of coffee later, our collaboration has deepened, and I am grateful for her perspective on life and research in Puebla. Several staff and faculty members at UPAEP helped with supporting this project with infrastructure, contacts, and logistics: Armando García Yáñez, Octavio González, Christelle Genestier, Liliana Rivadeneyra, Minerva Burelo, Paquita Castellanos, Elvira Carrillo, Doris Carrillo, Arturo Rojas, and Fátima Sierra. Finally, I want to thank Emilio Baños, the university's president, and José Pablo Nuño, the Director of Internationalization, who generously supported my work from the start.

I could not have done any of this work without the indefatigable energy of various student research assistants at the University of Notre Dame over the past few years. Becky Wornhoff, Amy Klopfenstein, Alexandria Christensen-Cabrera, Hannah Ray, Bernadette Miramontes, Sammie Escamilla, and Samuel Melgar contributed enormous amounts of time to helping with early data transcription and organization. For careful transcription of audio files, I especially want to thank Edna Martínez, Marina Pérez-Plazola, Rosa Mendoza, and Hannah Legatzke. Several students also read parts of the book's manuscript and provided thoughtful insights, comments, and critiques, which helped me to clarify my thoughts: Lauren O'Connell, Sara Berumen, Julia Mackessy, Marina Pérez-Plazola, George Timmins, Analie Fernandes, Katie Cox, Teagen Tibbot, Rachel Dinh, and Gigi Couri. The latter five were instrumental in helping with the bibliography, an enormous task. I am extremely grateful to anthropology PhD student Charles Morse, who spent many hours carefully creating a beautiful and detailed map of Puebla.

Three students accompanied me to Puebla and helped with data collection. Bernadette Miramontes and Edna Martínez accompanied me as freshmen in 2014 and 2016, respectively; they were great travel companions and very adept at finding people to interview. Megan Marshalla joined me in 2016 for an extended stay in Puebla as my research assistant and babysitter to my then five-year-old daughter. She excelled in both roles, and her love of sloths and patience with light shows will always remain with me. Her previous experiences in hospitals in Puebla and her own plans for attending medical school made her a truly unique research assistant. She quickly became invaluable; I greatly appreciate her willingness to be a sounding board for my plans. Her creativity, commitment, and good humor remained throughout her time in the field (even under sometimes difficult circumstances). I know she will make a wonderful physician one day.

I truly want to thank my friends and colleagues who unselfishly agreed to read early writings and manuscripts, and patiently listened to half-baked ideas. Carolyn Nordstrom, Jim Mckenna, and Agustín Fuentes always saw more in my work than I did, and they were supportive and inspiring throughout this research and writing, never flagging in their support. Friends and colleagues at Notre Dame, within anthropology and beyond, also gave moral and infrastructural support throughout this process: Sue Sheridan (whose bioarchaeology lab became a great place to write), Sarah McKibben, Vanesa Miseres, Donna Glowacki, Mark Golitko, Mark Schurr, Michelle Thornton, Eileen Barany, Rieti Gengo, and Marc Kissel. Gabriela Soto Laveaga's and Jaime Pensado's work on the historical medical/

student marches in Mexico inspired much of my analysis and interest in those of the present day. Carolyn Smith-Morris and Carole Browner provided sage advice on an early version of the prospectus. Claire Wendland read my conference papers, later carefully read more complete drafts, and provided thoughtful comments in person and through late-night e-mails. I am grateful for conversations and insights from my friends and colleagues within the anthropology of reproduction, especially Sarah Rubin, Mounia El Kotni, Eliza Williamson, and Dána-Ain Davis. Riikka Homanen and Miana Meskus's invitation to lecture at the University of Helsinki on early drafts about obstetric violence and gender in medicine helped me to strengthen my ideas substantially. I especially want to thank Lydia Dixon for her careful reading of several chapters and for providing insights into touch as well as the lack of touch. Her stunning work on the humanization of birth in Mexico inspired many of my ideas about obstetric violence. Beatriz Reyes-Foster has been hearing about this project for a long time, reading prospectuses and draft chapters, and was instrumental in introducing me to the editors at Rutgers and making a case for my book and my work. I am forever grateful.

I especially want to thank Kim Guinta, Editorial Director, and Lenore Manderson, Editor for the Medical Anthropology: Health, Inequality, and Social Justice Series at Rutgers University Press, who were both encouraging of the project and incredibly helpful and supportive as the book came into being. Lenore's incisive critiques helped me to revise and strengthen the manuscript before it went to press. Jasper Chang from Rutger's editorial department helped to keep me organized and on track. I know there were many people behind the scenes at Rutgers that helped to create this book; I am grateful to all of them. The two anonymous reviewers gave very thoughtful feedback that allowed me to solidify many of my ideas on medical selving; I am extremely grateful for the time and effort they put into reading the manuscript.

I owe a huge thank you to Mr. Hugo Saúl Ramírez Calderón and his brother Mr. Francisco Everardo Ramírez Calderón for their generosity in allowing me to use the image on the book's cover. The linocut, *Médico de Guardia* ("The Doctor's Office"), was made by their father, Maestro Everardo Ramírez Flores, from the Taller de Gráfica Popular in México in the mid-twentieth century. I was simply an unknown voice on the phone calling out of the blue to ask permission to reproduce the image on the cover. Without hesitation Mr. Hugo Ramírez gave his permission, asking nothing in return. I can never repay such kindness. I fell in love with the image during one of my classes at Notre Dame, where Bridget O'Brien Hoyt, the Curator of Education and Academic Programs at the Snite Museum of Art introduced my undergraduate students to the portrayal of medicine in art. Victoria Perdomo, Registrar at the Museum, was helpful in providing me access to an electronic copy of the image.

My most loving thanks goes to my family. It was because my sister Natalia lived in Puebla many years ago that this project even started; thank you for introducing me to *poblano* life. My sister Odette was patiently understanding of why I spent much of our family holiday staring at a screen rather than with the family. My parents, Pauline and Christopher, supported me generously throughout the years of this research—from logistics, to spending fun grandparent–granddaughter time, to feeding and housing me between Puebla trips. Through thick and thin my parents supported my writing of this book. When I felt I would never get the manuscript written, my mother urged me to just find a retreat and write until I was done; I followed her advice and, miraculously, managed to get to the end. My father was indefatigable in carefully reading every single chapter; in the process he caught many typos and gave me thoughtful feedback that helped me to rethink some of my arguments.

My daughter Kalpana and my husband Rahul, and our crazy four-legged feline and canine kin—Lucy, Gingerbread, Buñuelo, (and JellyBean)—are the heart and soul of my life. As a five-year-old, Kalpana spent part of her year in Puebla with me, attending kindergarten and loving every second of her stay. Her adaptability and keenness for her life there was contagious. Though I knew Puebla from my adult and researcher perspective, seeing the city through her eyes was transformative. Rahul's enthusiasm for my project was present from the beginning, materializing in long conversations about the practice and tragedy of medicine; his suggested framework of doctors as gods as well as the book's main title was just what I needed to make sense of all my data. Their patience and support for my writing was unparalleled. I love you all very much.

GLOSSARY

Casos clínicos: Clinical case presentations performed by medical trainees (interns or residents) as part of the learning process. They are sometimes known as grand rounds.

Compañero/a: Peers, work companions.

Guardia: Medical shift.

IMSS: The Mexican Institute for Social Security (Instituto Mexicano del Seguro Social), which provides medical care to workers of private companies, though this is not private insurance.

Intern: In Mexico, a medical student training at a hospital for one year during their fifth year of medical school.

ISSSTE: Security and Social Services for Workers of the State system (Instituto de Seguridad y Servicios Sociales de los Trabajadores del Estado), which provides medical care to workers of the state (teachers, police officers, other union workers).

Mestizo: Can refer to a person of mixed indigenous and European ancestry; the term has come to include cultural mixture as well.

Ministerio Público: The national jurisprudence and prosecutorial ministry.

Pasante: In Mexico, a physician serving a mandatory year of social service providing medical care to rural or underserved communities after completing their internship.

Poblano/a: It has multiple meanings: someone who resides in the city of Puebla; someone who descends from Spanish colonizers; and, at times, people elsewhere in Mexico use it to stereotype poblanos as conservative, classist, elitist, or parochial.

Resident: In Mexico, a physician who has passed the national residency examination and is training for a specialty at a hospital.

Scrubs: Protective and sanitary clothing (usually shirt and trousers) designed to be worn by physicians, nurses, and other medical personnel within surgeries.

Secretaría de Salud: The Ministry of Health.

NOTES

INTRODUCTION

1. Scrubs are part of the uniform for medical workers. In Mexico these are called *piyama quirúrgica*—surgical pajama—which evinces their simplicity, sterility, and comfort. Doctors in my field sites tended to almost exclusively wear these in sterile spaces or during overnight shifts, though in other countries they might also be used as part of the daily uniform.

2. The convention in these hospitals was that only attending physicians were called by their title and last name (e.g., Doctor Contreras) while residents were called by their title and first name (e.g., Doctora Valentina). I followed these formal conventions in my interactions with the doctors during my research and have employed them in this book. However, though interns were often called by the title of doctor and their first name, because of the closeness of my interactions with them I have chosen to use their first names here. Regardless of whom I am writing about, I have used a pseudonym for all people's names and most places, unless otherwise noted and have sometimes hidden identifying characteristics to protect my interlocutors' identity.

3. Each year approximately 50,000 applicants take the national residency examination, of which fewer than 10 percent pass.

4. The government measures "indigeneity" on the national census based on people's self-reported use of an Indigenous language. In the state of Puebla, 11 percent of people speak an Indigenous language.

5. The Ministry of Health was subsequently reformed and renamed in 1943 and 1982.

6. By the turn of the twenty-first century, the IMSS was the largest social service institution in Latin America.

7. Whereby *popular* can dually translate as Popular or People's Health Insurance. It provided approximately half the country's population access to 290 essential and sixty-five high-cost interventions (Frenk, Gómez-Dantés, and Knaul 2019).

8. Known by his initials, AMLO. Although far-left in his rhetoric, many of his policies have paradoxically been decidedly unleftist, such as austerity measures and drastically reducing expenditure toward education and social welfare.

9. The state of Puebla has a ratio of almost six hospitals per 100,000 people, ranking eighth in the nation—though most of these hospitals are in the city of Puebla (Secretaría de Salud 2016).

10. The average total cost for attending a public medical school is $2,238 and for a private school it is $58,594 (IMCO 2018). Most private schools offer need-based scholarships.

11. The Mexican average monthly salary for 2020 was just under $300 dollars. The daily minimum wage was 123.22 pesos ($5.5 dollars).

12. This same study indicated that the fathers of these children worked in the following professions: professional (30 percent), administration (21.3 percent), merchants (13.8 percent), and laborers (13.3 percent), while their mothers worked as professionals (20.3 percent), administrators (14.8 percent), and as homemakers (41.1 percent).

13. The human development index (HDI), a summary measure of various factors (i.e., life expectancy, education, and per capita income), is used to rank countries regarding their human development. Some of Puebla's municipalities have HDIs similar to countries like Uruguay or Serbia, and others have HDIs more similar to Haiti.

14. In U.S. dollars, these wages translate to approximately $6.57 and $2.15 a day, respectively (Consejo Nacional de Evaluación de la Política de Desarrollo Social [CONEVAL] 2015).

15. "Prepare" (*prepárate*) was a play on words achieved by splitting the word into two: prepare (*preparar*) and stand (*parar*).

16. According to data from the Ministry of Health (Secretaría de Salud 2016), the largest proportion of cesarean deliveries occur in the private sector (77 percent), followed by ISSSTE hospitals (68 percent); the lowest occur in IMSS hospitals, with an average of 25 percent. All of these are well above the 10 percent to 15 percent recommended by the World Health Organization. Puebla ranks eleventh highest nationwide.

1. WOMEN CAN'T BE TRAUMA DOCTORS

1. In some of my translations, I also include the original Spanish word(s). If part of the meaning is lost in translation, I include the Spanish for context. Or if there is an expression that conveys a more grounded, local meaning, I keep it in.

2. These perceptions were not simply held by men and used to disenfranchise their female colleagues. My female interlocutors held two distinct and contradictory sets of beliefs: they stated that, overall, women were prone to weakness and hysteria, while they simultaneously rebelled against perceptions that *they* were personally not as competent as men.

3. Gender in these spaces was binary. All my interlocutors self-identified as cis-gender. I occasionally heard pejorative comments that emphasized a particular worldview and way of being that left little space for the nonbinary "other."

4. Then-president Porfirio Díaz provided permission, even attending Montoya's graduation in person.

5. These comments are similar to the now-discredited statements of Harvard University president Edward Clarke who, in a speech in 1873, claimed that when women were educated all their blood and energy went to their brain, atrophying their reproductive organs so the women became "neuralgic and hysterical" (Clarke 1884, 84); he believed engaging in nonfeminine labor would change women's physiology and maternal instincts, making them coarse and deviant (92).

6. By providing health and charitable care to the population, hospital care was a strategy used by the church to increase its power (Fajardo-Ortíz 1999).

7. The Real y Pontificia Universidad de México (Royal and Pontifical University of Mexico) was nationalized and liberalized centuries later, becoming the National Autonomous University of Mexico, the UNAM (Rodríguez 2010).

8. Beatriz Reyes-Foster (2018) provides a thorough examination of the nuances present in identity and mestizaje in Mexico and how these shape people's experiences in medical care.

9. During most of the mid- to late-nineteenth century the president was Porfirio Díaz, who served for seven terms and a total of more than thirty years. His long dictatorship and multiple re-elections, in part, catalyzed the 1910 Mexican Revolution. As expected, Díaz is a controversial character in history. He ushered in a scientific and positivist view into society, education, and politics, modernizing the country through the building of railways connecting urban centers and ports. But there was also a marked increase in the social and economic disparities between the country's population.

10. The day the first "modern" medical school was inaugurated (October 23) is now annually commemorated as the *Día del Médico*—Doctors' Day—by medical schools and practitioners across Mexico, celebrating what is considered to be the official beginning of Mexican biomedicine.

11. Many governing bodies regulate medicine (the Ministry of Education, the Mexican Association of Medical Colleges and Schools, the National Association of Universities and Institutes for Higher Education, etc.). These do not always have the same standards, and not all medical schools are accredited and monitored.

12. The rest of the country sometimes stereotypes poblanos as classist and elitist.

13. He examined the hymens of 181 women to identify which was the most common shape, arguing that this information would best protect female virginity and, consequently, the country's morality (Ruiz 2001).

14. In 1977 the original maternity hospital was converted into a teaching hospital for students at a private medical school affiliated with Hospital Piedad.

15. I have used the term *Rosa Salvaje,* which was the title of a highly successful telenovela in Mexico in the 1980s. Because I use pseudonyms, I created a pseudonym that was close enough to "Rosa's" actual name in order for the resident's comment to make sense.

16. According to Cassell, female surgeons cannot humiliate their students in the same way as male physicians, or people would complain.

2. DOCTORS ON THE MARCH

1. Perhaps it is indicative of how much I had been accepted by them that I was included in their backstage humor.

2. An otorhinolaryngology surgeon is an ears, nose, and throat/head and neck surgeon.

3. Two parallel forces were occurring—on the one hand, the rapid expansion of the health institutes, and on the other the effort to make medical training more rigorous and more standardized, particularly emulating the U.S. system of medical training.

4. It began at the Hospital 20 de Noviembre, so named for the start date of the Mexican Revolution.

5. One source stated that the IMSS hospital where the patients from the damaged hospital were moved originally had 178 beds; it was increased to 253, although their population base had almost tripled (almost a million and a half patients). By December 2019 it was meant to have 310 beds, in addition to a planned 100-bed obstetrics wing to increase the number of beds to just over 400 by mid-2021 (Aroche 2019).

6. I followed Mexican convention about formality of address and used "usted" for all residents, attending physicians, and nurses (and other staff), while using the more informal "tú" with my direct interlocutors, the interns. Although I was several years older than the residents and my age should have made me "senior" to them, not one of them invited me to use the informal form of address. I can only conclude that their rank was above mine in these spaces. I had the reverse situation with the interns, who clearly saw me as an old professor; most (but, fortunately, not all) used "usted" despite my entreaties to be more informal.

7. The names and ranks of the sixteen doctors are not public knowledge, although given the structure of medical care in public hospitals, it is likely that many were trainees.

8. The boy's father demanded an investigation, performed by the National Commission for Medical Arbitration (CONAMED). The commission concluded that there was bad praxis but not medical negligence (though the later arrest warrants did accuse the doctors of medical negligence).

9. On Twitter, the search URL https://twitter.com/hashtag/YoSoy17?src=hash will pull up many protest tweets. The protest's name was likely inspired by an earlier political campaign called #YoSoy132, which was a response in 2012 to the election of Enrique Peña Nieto as the country's president.

10. One of the communiqués of the protesters blamed the "neoliberal assault" on health-care institutions, which cared more about decreasing costs than about investing in infrastructure, equipment, or medical training. They blamed the government for enrolling patients into health programs such as Seguro Popular rather than making sure the health institutions were equipped to care for them. These conditions created the high patient load wherein clinicians and hospitals were stretched to capacity. The communiqué further stated that there were asymmetries in the quality of services that hospitals could provide and in the distribution of clinicians within hospitals and across the nation (too many in urban, not enough in rural), and a lack of incentives for clinicians to work in underserved areas. They further reminded the public that no sane doctor would wish to harm their patient and that the trust of patients toward their doctors is sacred (a concept repeatedly told to me by participants). The document further argued that the state needed to provide the proper and optimal conditions for the doctor–patient relationship to be successful. The insecurity and violence for doctors across the nation made their sacrifice even more marked. Finally, they added that the legal repercussions to medical mistakes undermined their professional identity. The full communiqué was posted on the group's Facebook page.

11. His plan was criticized by patients and doctors, with calls for clarity about what conditions would be covered and how patients would recover their costs for tertiary and specialized care. The six most recent ministers of health said it was a serious mistake to cancel Seguro Popular, which, they claimed, was "one of the most important institutional advances" the country had made in several decades.

3. THE SOUL OF THE HOSPITAL

1. Students take an entrance examination for university (specific to each university).

2. Interns have a higher workload in hospitals where there is a lack of staff and a higher patient load, such as at many of the public hospitals in Mexico, and a lower load at smaller hospitals and private ones.

3. Scrub technicians (or scrub techs) are some of the first surgery team members to enter into the sterile space, scrubbing in first, laying out the instruments, and setting up the sterile drapes (in conjunction with surgical nurses). They dress the surgeons and team members in gowns and gloves. During the surgery they pass the instruments and supplies to the surgery team, monitoring what supplies are used. In Mexico it is considered one of the main parts of training during an intern's rotation in any surgical specialty.

4. At most hospitals trainees are divided into three groups (called A, B, and C) and carry out their guardia with their assigned group. In 2018, guardias were spaced out into no more than twice a week.

5. Tenckhoff catheters are inserted into the abdominal cavity and are usually used for drainage. Subclavian catheters (central line catheters) are inserted into a large vein in the upper torso.

6. Medical evidence suggests that controlled cord traction can sometimes reduce the risk of postpartum hemorrhage if used in conjunction with uterotonic medications.

4. INTERNALIZING AND REPRODUCING VIOLENCE

1. Some sources suggest that the death rate is higher but that they are not identified as femicides because they lack evidence of gendered violence (Nájar 2017) or because they are "black rates" (*cifras negras*), defined as the number of crimes or delinquents whose crimes have

either not been reported by their victims or they have not been discovered by the system (Pérez Oseguera and Espíndola Pérez 2015).

2. In November 2014, forty-three student-teachers from Ayotzinapa, in the state of Guerrero, were disappeared (and likely killed) by drug cartels, which marked one of the lowest points in the country's drug-related violence. Since 2007, tens of thousands of people have been killed, and several thousand more have been forcibly disappeared.

3. Reports show that Mara also had used these hashtags a few months before she was murdered. Based on Ni Una Menos, an Argentine feminist movement against gender-based violence, ¡Ni Una Mas! was formed in Mexico for the same purpose.

4. Because the violence has not diminished, these marches continue to occur. One of the most recent was on March 8–9, 2020 (coinciding with International Women's Day), a massive strike where thousands of women marched with the slogans of #UnDíaSinNosotras (#ADayWithoutUs) and #UnDíaSinMujeres (#ADayWithoutWomen).

5. Efforts were made to urge the Puebla state government to issue a gender alert, which was ultimately rejected (Instituto Nacional de las Mujeres [Inmujeres] 2018).

6. The average fetal heart rate is between 110 and 160 beats per minute.

7. Misoprostol began its pharmaceutical life as a treatment for stomach ulcers. It was later discovered to have unintended side effects on uterine contractions and cervical dilations. It is used worldwide to induce labor and for legal and illicit abortions.

8. Merthiolate is widely used for antiseptic purposes.

9. Hospital Piedad has a cesarean rate of approximately 95 percent, a rate not uncommon in private hospitals in Mexico (Soto-Vega et al. 2015). Additionally, the percentage of births attended in biomedical settings rose from 72.6 percent to 80.0 percent between 2005 and 2008 (Programa de las Naciones Unidas para el Desarrollo [PNUD] 2014).

10. Claire Wendland, personal communication, January 14, 2020. The "easiest" fetal presentation is occiput anterior (head down and the body facing toward the mother's back) because the baby's head has a smoother fit through the pelvis. Right occiput transverse babies sometimes rotate to occiput posterior, which can be a longer and more painful labor, though not impossible to birth vaginally. According to Claire Wendland (personal communication), "vaginal delivery isn't always impossible for an [occiput transverse] baby, but it's quite difficult" because of the mismatch between fetal dimensions and pelvic dimensions and because it is hard for the fetus to "rotate through the usual movements necessary for descending through the pelvis." Skilled doctors can potentially "push the fetal head up out of the pelvis and flex it; when it comes down again, it'll naturally rotate into an [occiput anterior] position." Another option is a forceps rotation, which can also take significant skill. In our conversation, Wendland added that because of the deskilling of physicians, many of these lower-technology approaches are not considered. Work by Shetty et al. (2014) showed that vaginal examination was remarkably inaccurate in determining fetal head position (about 30 percent accuracy).

11. Engagement means that the baby's head has descended to where the widest part of its diameter has passed the midpoint of the mother's pelvis.

12. Though I aided the interns and residents in supporting Miranda, the better support would have been from someone she knew and trusted.

13. Claire Wendland, personal communication, 2020.

14. The pubic symphysis is a cartilaginous joint at the lower end of the pubic bones, just below the bladder. Uterine inversion means when the uterus turns inside out; it can be caused by pulling on the umbilical cord or by manual fundal pressure (pushing on the top of the uterus) before the placenta has detached.

15. Like other medical interventions, this technique should be carried out only when absolutely necessary as it can be lifesaving under some circumstances when the placenta breaks apart (Perlman and Carusi 2019).

16. Cephalohematomas are bruising or swelling under the skin of the parietal region of the cranium.

5. THE BODY LEARNS

Note: Parts of the data in this chapter appear in my article (coauthored with Megan Marshalla) in *American Anthropologist* (2019), though the analysis and discussion are very different in each publication.

1. Almost all the surgeries I attended had music playing. The space belongs to the surgeons, and they make it theirs through choosing the type of music that will play; they usually bring in a phone with playlists.

2. The Spanish *óbito* comes from the Latin *obitus,* meaning "death" or "perished." It is the same root word used for obituary.

3. Lydia Dixon (personal communication, May 2019) stated that the midwifery students in her research in central Mexico also "went through life measuring everything with their two fingers."

4. On the surface these seem to be different phrases (*meter mano:* put your hands into [something]; and *hacer manitas:* be handy). However, I use them interchangeably in the same way as my interlocutors did.

5. A partogram shows key maternal and fetal data (cervical dilation, fetal heart rate, vital signs, etc.) during labor graphically represented against time.

6. An underactive thyroid can cause the body's metabolism to slow down. It can affect a woman's ability to become pregnant or can cause miscarriage.

7. I described this procedure in chapter 3 during Wendy's mistake with the cord avulsion.

8. Interestingly, the clinicians' treatment of Cleo is kinder than most medical interactions I and other scholars have witnessed in Mexico—she is spoken to by name, they talk gently to her when they have her hold her baby, and they ask her permission to take the baby to prepare it for the morgue.

9. Uterine tone refers to the muscle tone of the uterus. A normal uterus will contract during labor, compressing the blood vessels. If the contractions are not strong enough there is a greater risk of hemorrhage.

10. I elaborate on this birth in other writings, focusing on the obstetrically violent parts of this procedure, including the ways that Graciela was pressured to undergo a tubal ligation immediately after her cesarean.

11. This pressing action is referred to as manual fundal pressure, widely considered to be obstetrically violent because it is painful and might result in morbidities to the mother and baby (World Health Organization 2018b).

REFERENCES

Adams, Tracey L. 2010. "Gender and Feminization in Health Care Professions." *Sociology Compass* 4 (7): 454–465.

Agostoni, Claudia. 2003. *Monuments of Progress: Modernization and Public Health in Mexico City, 1876–1910*. Calgary: University of Calgary Press.

———. 2007. "La Salud Pública durante el México Porfiriano (1876–1910)." In *Historia de la Medicina en México,* edited by Carlos Viesca, 247–257. Mexico City: Universidad Nacional Autónoma de México.

Aguilar, Rosario. 2013. "Los Tonos de los Desafíos Democráticos: El Color de la Piel y la Raza en México." In "Desafíos de la Política Mexicana," edited by Elizabeth J. Zechmeister. Thematic Volume, *Política y Gobierno,* 25–57.

Ahmed, Sara. 2012. *On Being Included: Racism and Diversity in Institutional Life.* Durham, NC: Duke University Press.

Allahyari, Rebecca A. 1996. "'Ambassadors of God' and 'The Sinking Classes': Visions of Charity and Moral Selving." *International Journal of Sociology and Social Policy* 16 (1/2): 35–69.

———. 2000. *Visions of Charity: Volunteer Workers and Moral Community.* Berkeley: University of California Press.

Amnistía Internacional. 2020. "Global: Análisis de Amnistía Internacional Revela que Más de 7 Mil Personas Trabajadoras de la Salud Han Muerto a Causa de COVID-19." https://amnistia.org.mx/contenido/index.php/global-analisis-de-amnistia-internacional-revela-que-mas-de-7-mil-personas-trabajadoras-de-la-salud-han-muerto-a-causa-de-covid-19/.

Andaya, Elise. 2019. "Race-ing Time: Clinical Temporalities and Inequality in Public Prenatal Care." *Medical Anthropology* 38 (8): 651–663.

Anderson, Nancy, and Michael Dietrich. 2012. *The Educated Eye: Visual Culture and Pedagogy in the Life Sciences.* Lebanon, NH: Dartmouth College Press.

Anderson, Warwick. 2009. "Modern Sentinel and Colonial Microcosm: Science, Discipline, and Distress at the Philippine General Hospital." *Philippine Studies* 57 (2): 153–177.

Archundia-García, Abel. 2011. "El Movimiento Médico en 1964–1965." *Revista de Especialidades Médico-Quirúrgicas* 16 (S1): S28–S31.

Arias Amaral, Jaime, and María G. Ramos Ponce. 2011. "Mujer y Medicina: La Historia de Matilde Petra Montoya Lafragua." *Medicina Interna de México* 27 (5): 467–469.

Aristegui Noticias. 2014. "Somos Médicos, No Somos Criminales, Marcha Histórica #YoSoy17, en Más de 20 Estados." *Aristegui Noticias,* June 23, 2014. http://aristeguinoticias.com/2306/mexico/somos-medicos-no-somos-criminales-marcha-historica-yosoy17-en-mas-de-20-estados/.

Aroche, Ernesto. 2019. "Fallido Proyecto de Nuevo Hospital Satura de Servicios del IMSS en Puebla." *Animal Político,* October 10. https://www.animalpolitico.com/2019/10/fallido-proyecto-hospital-saturacion-imss-puebla/.

Auyero, Javier. 2012. *Patients of the State: The Politics of Waiting in Argentina.* Durham, NC: Duke University Press.

Babaria, Palav, Sakena Abedin, David Berg, and Marcella Nunez-Smith. 2012. "'I'm Too Used to It': A Longitudinal Qualitative Study of Third Year Female Medical Students' Experiences of Gendered Encounters in Medical Education." *Social Science and Medicine* 74 (7): 1013–1020.

Barthelemy, Ramón S., Melinda McCormick, and Charles Henderson. 2016. "Gender Discrimination in Physics and Astronomy: Graduate Student Experiences of Sexism and Gender Microaggressions." *Physical Review Physics Education Research* 12 (2): 020119.

Beagan, Brenda L. 2000. "Neutralizing Differences: Producing Neutral Doctors for (Almost) Neutral Patients." *Social Science and Medicine* 51 (8): 1253–1265.

Bennett, Linda Rae, and Bregje de Kok. 2018. "Reproductive Desires and Disappointments." *Medical Anthropology* 37 (2): 91–100.

Berg, Marc, and Geoffrey Bowker. 1997. "The Multiple Bodies of the Medical Record: Toward a Sociology of an Artifact." *Sociological Quarterly* 38:513–537.

Bhagwati, Anuradha. 2019. *Unbecoming: A Memoir of Disobedience.* New York: Atria Books.

Biehl, João, Byron Good, and Arthur Kleinman, eds. 2007. *Subjectivity: Ethnographic Investigations.* Berkeley: University of California Press.

Biswas, Shampa. 2019. "Advice on Advising: How to Mentor Minority Students." *Chronicle of Higher Education,* March 13, 2019. https://www.chronicle.com/article/Advice-on-Advising-How-to/245870.

Blanch, Danielle C., Judith A. Hall, Debra L. Roter, and Richard M. Frankel. 2008. "Medical Student Gender and Issues of Confidence." *Patient Education and Counseling* 72 (3): 374–381.

Bolton, Sharon, and Daniel Muzio. 2008. "The Paradoxical Processes of Feminization in the Professions: The Case of Established, Aspiring and Semi-Professions." *Work, Employment and Society* 22 (2): 281–299.

Bosk, Charles L. 2003. *Forgive and Remember: Managing Medical Failure.* 2nd ed. Chicago: University of Chicago Press.

Bourdieu, Pierre. (1977) 2000. *Outline of a Theory of Practice.* Cambridge: Cambridge University Press.

Bourdieu, Pierre, and Loïc J. D. Wacquant. 1992. *An Invitation to Reflexive Sociology.* Chicago: University of Chicago Press.

Braff, Lara. 2013. "Somos Muchos (We Are So Many): Population Politics and 'Reproductive Othering' in Mexican Fertility Clinics." *Medical Anthropology Quarterly* 27 (1): 121–138.

Brandes, Stanley. 2002. "Drink, Abstinence, and Male Identity in Mexico City." In *Changing Men and Masculinities in Latin America,* edited by Matthew C. Gutmann, 153–178. Durham, NC: Duke University Press.

Briceño Morales, Ximena, Laura V. Enciso Chaves, and Carlos E. Yepes Delgado. 2018. "Neither Medicine nor Health Care Staff Members Are Violent by Nature: Obstetric Violence from an Interactionist Perspective." *Qualitative Health Research* 28 (8): 1308–1319.

Bridges, Khiara M. 2011. *Reproducing Race: An Ethnography of Pregnancy as a Site of Racialization.* Berkeley: University of California Press.

Briggs, Laura. 2000. "The Race of Hysteria: 'Overcivilization' and the 'Savage' Woman in Late Nineteenth-Century Obstetrics and Gynecology." *American Quarterly* 52 (2): 246–273.

Briseño, Héctor. 2020. "Médicos Protestan en Acapulco por Asesinato de Directora de Hospital." *La Jornada,* August 1, 2020. https://www.jornada.com.mx/ultimas/estados/2020/08/01/medicos-protestan-en-acapulco-por-asesinato-de-directora-de-hospital-4647.html.

Brown, Mike. 2017. "The Offshore Sailor: Enskilment and Identity," *Leisure Studies* 36 (5): 684–695.

Bruce, Adrienne N., Alexis Battista, Michael W. Plankey, Lynt B. Johnson, and M. Blair Marshall. 2015. "Perceptions of Gender-based Discrimination During Surgical Training and Practice." *Medical Education Online* 20:25923.

Butler, Judith. 1993. *Bodies That Matter: On the Discursive Limits of Sex.* New York: Routledge.

Cabello-López, Alejandro, Rodrigo Gopar-Nieto, Guadalupe Aguilar-Madrid, Cuauhtémoc A. Juárez-Pérez, and Luis C. Haro-García. 2015. "Perspectiva Histórica y Social del Movimiento Médico de 1964–1965 en México." *Revista Médica del Instituto Mexicano del Seguro Social* 53 (4): 466–471.

Calabrese, Joseph D. 2011. "'The Culture of Medicine' As Revealed in Patients' Perspectives on Psychiatric Treatment. In *Shattering Culture: American Medicine Responds to Cultural Diversity*, edited by Mary-Jo D. Good, Sarah S. Willen, Seth Donal Hannah, Ken Vickery, and Lawrence Taeseng Park, 184–199. New York: Russell Sage Foundation.

Camacho Servín, Fernando. 2020. "Quitarse el Miedo, Primer Paso de Médicos contra el Covid. *La Jornada*, August 3, 2020. https://www.jornada.com.mx/ultimas/politica/2020/08/03/quitarse-el-miedo-primer-paso-de-medicos-contra-el-covid-3113.html.

Camacho-Villarreal, A. L., and J. C. Pérez-López. 2013. "Revisión de Cavidad Uterina Instrumentada Gentil Frente a la Revisión Manual y su Relación con la Hemorragia Posparto." *Enfermería Universitaria* 10 (1): 21–26.

Camhaji, Alías, and Almudena Barragán. 2017. "Mara no se Fue, a Mara la Mataron." *El País*, September 18, 2017. https://elpais.com/internacional/2017/09/17/mexico/1505666780_800518.html.

Carpenter-Song, Elizabeth. 2011. "Recognition in Clinical Relationships". In *Shattering Culture: American Medicine Responds to Cultural Diversity*, edited by Mary-Jo D. Good, Sarah S. Willen, Seth Donal Hannah, Ken Vickery, and Lawrence Taeseng Park, 168–183. New York: Russell Sage Foundation.

Carrillo-Esper, Raúl, Teresa de la Torre-León, Isis Espinoza-de los Monteros, and Dulce María Carrillo-Córdova. 2015. "Matilde Petra Montoya Lafragua. Breve Historia de una Mexicana Ejemplar." *Revista Mexicana de Anestesiología* 38 (3): 161–165.

Casas-Patiño, Donovan, Sergio Reséndiz-Rivera, and Isaac Casas. 2009. "Reseña Cronológica del Movimiento Médico 1964–1965." *Boletín Mexicano de Historia y Filosofía de la Medicina* 12 (1): 9–13.

Casas-Patiño, Donovan, Alejandra Rodríguez Torres, Isaac Casas-Patiño, and Cuauhtémoc Galeana Castillo. 2013. "Médicos Residentes en México: Tradición o Humillación." *Medwave* 13 (7): e5764.

Cassell, Joan. 1997. "Doing Gender, Doing Surgery: Women Surgeons in a Man's Profession." *Human Organization* 56 (1): 47–52.

———. 2000. *The Woman in the Surgeon's Body.* Cambridge, MA: Harvard University Press.

Castillo, Kara. 2018. "A un Año del Sismo, Saturación de Urgencias de la Margarita, un Problema de Salud Pública." *La Jornada de Oriente,* September 19, 2018. https://www.lajornadadeoriente.com.mx/puebla/a-un-ano-del-sismo-saturacion-de-urgencias-de-la-margarita-un-problema-de-salud-publica/.

Castillo Yáñez, Lizbeth. 2016. "Médicos de la Ciudad de México Realizarán Marcha a las 16 Horas." *Saludiario.* June 22, 2016. http://saludiario.com/medicos-de-la-ciudad-de-mexico-realizaran-marcha-a-las-16-horas/.

Castro, Arachu, and Virginia Savage. 2019. "Obstetric Violence as Reproductive Governance in the Dominican Republic." *Medical Anthropology* 38 (2): 123–136.

Castro, Roberto. 2014. "Génesis y Práctica del Habitus Médico Autoritario en México." *Revista Mexicana de Sociología* 76 (2): 167–197.

Castro, Roberto, and Joaquina Erviti. 2014. "25 Años de Investigación sobre Violencia Obstétrica en México." *Revista CONAMED* 19 (1): 37–42.

Castro, Roberto, and Sonia M. Frías. 2019. "Obstetric Violence in Mexico: Results from a 2016 National Household Survey." *Violence against Women* 26 (6–7): 555–572.

Castro, Roberto, and Marcia Villanueva Lozano. 2018. "Violencia en la Práctica Médica en México: Un Caso de Ambivalencia Sociológica." *Estudios Sociológicos* 36 (108): 539–569.

Castro Morales, Efraín. 2009. "La Escuela de Medicina de Puebla." *Tiempo Universitario* 12 (8): 1–8.

Chatburn, Alex, Mark J. Kohler, Jessica D. Payne, and Sean P. A. Drummond. 2017. "The Effects of Sleep Restriction and Sleep Deprivation in Producing False Memories." *Neurobiology of Learning and Memory* 137: 107–113.

Clancy, Kathryn B. H., Robin G. Nelson, Julienne N. Rutherford, and Katie Hinde. 2014. "Survey of Academic Field Experiences (SAFE): Trainees Report Harassment and Assault." *PLOS One* 9 (7): e102172.

Clarke, Edward H. 1884. *Sex in Education; A Fair Chance for Girls.* Boston: Houghton Mifflin.

Colas, Kelly. 2017. "Reproducing Inequality: An Examination of Physician Decision-Making During Childbirth in Merida, Mexico." PhD diss., Michigan State University.

Colen, Shellee. 1995. "'Like a Mother to Them': Stratified Reproduction and West Indian Childcare Workers and Employers in New York." In *Conceiving the New World Order: The Global Politics of Reproduction,* edited by Faye D. Ginsburg and Rayna Rapp, 78–102. Berkeley: University of California Press.

Comisión de Derechos Humanos del Estado de Puebla (CDHP). 2015. "Recomendación Número: 3/2015, Expediente: 8943/2013-C De Oficio a Favor de Médicos Residentes Adscritos a las Instituciones que Integran el Sistema Nacional de Salud." http://www.cdhpuebla.org.mx/pdf/Rec/15/3-2015.pdf.

Consejo, Carolina, and Carlos Viesca-Treviño. 2008. "Ética y Relaciones de Poder en la Formación de Médicos Residentes e Internos: Algunas Reflexiones a la Luz de Foucault y Bourdieu." *Boletín Mexicano de Historia y Filosofía de la Medicina* 11 (1): 16–20.

Consejo Nacional de Evaluación de la Política de Desarrollo Social (CONEVAL). 2015. "Entidades Federativas, Pobreza a Nivel Municipio 2015: Puebla." https://www.coneval.org.mx/coordinacion/entidades/Puebla/Paginas/pobreza_municipal2015.aspx.

Cornwall, Andrea, and Nancy Lindisfarne, eds. 1994. *Dislocating Masculinity: Comparative Ethnographies.* London: Routledge.

Cortés-Flores, Ana O., Clotilde Fuentes-Orozco, María K. L. López-Ramírez, Gabriela A. Velázquez-Ramírez, Oscar A. Farías-Llamas, Juan J. Olivares-Becerra, and Alejandro González-Ojeda. 2005. "Medicina Académica y Género: La Mujer en Especialidades Quirúrgicas." *Gaceta Médica de México* 141 (4): 341–344.

Coser, Rose L. 1962. *Life in the Ward.* East Lansing: Michigan State University Press.

Criado-Perez, Caroline. 2019. "The Deadly Truth about a World Built for Men—From Stab Vests to Car Crashes." *The Guardian,* February 23, 2019. https://www.theguardian.com/lifeandstyle/2019/feb/23/truth-world-built-for-men-car-crashes.

Crowley-Matoka, Megan. 2016. *Domesticating Organ Transplant: Familial Sacrifice and National Aspiration in Mexico.* Durham, NC: Duke University Press.

Cruz Bárcenas, Arturo. 2015. La Sicología del Poblano, Consecuencia de su Realidad Histórica y Social. *La Jornada,* May 29, 2015. https://www.jornada.com.mx/2015/05/29/espectaculos/a10n1esp.

Csordas, Thomas J. 1990. "Embodiment as a Paradigm for Anthropology." *Ethos* 18 (1): 5–47.

———. 1993. "Somatic Modes of Attention." *Cultural Anthropology* 8 (2): 135–156.

Cuarón, Alfonso, dir. 2018. *Roma.* Mexico City: Esperanto Filmoj.

Datos Abiertos. 2016. *Personal Médico por Municipio del ISSSTEP.* http://datos.puebla.gob.mx/datasetpersonal-medico-municipio-issstep.

Davies, Celia. 1996. "The Sociology of Professions and the Profession of Gender." *Sociology* 30 (4): 661–678.

Davis, Dána-Ain. 2019a. "Obstetric Racism: The Racial Politics of Pregnancy, Labor, and Birthing." *Medical Anthropology* 38 (7): 560–573.

———. 2019b. *Reproductive Injustice: Racism, Pregnancy, and Premature Birth*. New York: New York University Press.

Davis, Dána-Ain, and Christa Craven. 2016. *Feminist Ethnography: Thinking through Methodologies, Challenges, and Possibilities*. Lanham, MD: Rowman & Littlefield.

Davis, Georgiann, and Rachel Allison. 2013. "Increasing Representation, Maintaining Hierarchy: An Assessment of Gender and Medical Specialization." *Social Thought and Research* 32:17–45.

Davis-Floyd, Robbie E. 1994. "The Technocratic Body: American Childbirth as Cultural Expression." *Social Science and Medicine* 38 (8): 1125–1140.

———. 2003. *Birth as an American Rite of Passage: With a New Preface*. Berkeley: University of California Press.

De la Garza-Aguilar, Javier. 2005. "Reflexiones sobre la Calidad de la Carrera de Medicina en México." *Gaceta Médica de México* 141 (2): 129–141.

De López, Jenna M. 2018. "When the Scars Begin to Heal: Narratives of Obstetric Violence in Chiapas, Mexico." *International Journal of Health Governance* 23 (1): 60–69.

Demaiter, Erin I., and Tracey L. Adams. 2009. "'I Really Didn't Have Any Problems with the Male-Female Thing Until . . .': Successful Women's Experiences in IT Organizations." *Canadian Journal of Sociology* 34 (1): 31–53.

Derive, Stephanie, María de la Luz Casas-Martínez, Gregorio T. Obrador Vera, Antonio R. Villa, and Daniela Contreras. 2018. "Percepción de Maltrato Durante la Residencia Médica en México: Medición y Análisis Bioético." *Investigación en Educación Médica* 7 (26): 35–44.

Díaz-Portillo, Sandra P., Álvaro J. Idrovo, Anahí Dreser, Federico R. Bonilla, Bonifacia Matías-Juan, and Veronika J. Wirtz. 2015. "Consultorios Adyacentes a Farmacias Privadas en México: Infraestructura y Características del Personal Médico y su Remuneración." *Salud Pública de México* 57 (4): 320–328.

Diniz, Simone G., and Alessandra S. Chacham. 2004. "'The Cut Above' and 'The Cut Below': The Abuse of Caesareans and Episiotomy in São Paulo, Brazil." *Reproductive Health Matters* 12 (23): 100–110.

Dixon, Lydia Z. 2020. *Delivering Health: Midwifery and Development in Mexico*. Nashville, TN: Vanderbilt University Press.

Dixon, Lydia Zacher. 2015 "Obstetrics in a Time of Violence: Mexican Midwives Critique Routine Hospital Practices." *Medical Anthropology Quarterly* 29 (4): 437–454.

Dixon, Lydia Zacher, Vania Smith-Oka, and Mounia El Kotni. 2019. "Teaching about Childbirth in Mexico: Working across Birth Models." In *Birth in Eight Cultures*, edited by Robbie Davis-Floyd and Melissa Cheney, 17–47. Long Grove, IL: Waveland Press.

Dore, Elizabeth. 2000. "One Step Forward, Two Steps Back: Gender and the State in the Long Nineteenth Century." In *Hidden Histories of Gender and the State in Latin America*, edited by Elizabeth Dore and Maxine Molyneux, 3–32. Durham, NC: Duke University Press.

Downey, Greg. 2010. "'Practice without Theory': A Neuroanthropological Perspective on Embodied Learning." *Journal of the Royal Anthropological Institute* 16 (S1): S22–S40.

Draper, Jan. 2002. "'It was a Real Good Show': The Ultrasound Scan, Fathers and the Power of Visual Knowledge." *Sociology of Health and Illness* 24 (6): 771–795.

Dreyfus, Hubert. 1992. *What Computers Still Can't Do: A Critique of Artificial Reason*. Cambridge, MA: MIT Press.

Dulitzky, Ariel E. 2005. "A Region in Denial: Racial Discrimination and Racism in Latin America." In *Neither Enemies nor Friends: Latinos, Blacks, and Afro-Latinos*, edited by Anani Dzidzienyo and Suzanne Oboler, 39–59. New York: Palgrave Macmillan.

Duncan, Whitney L. 2017. "Psicoeducación in the Land of Magical Thoughts: Culture and Mental-Health Practice in a Changing Oaxaca." *American Ethnologist* 44 (1): 36–51.

———. 2018. *Transforming Therapy: Mental Health Practice and Cultural Change in Mexico.* Nashville, TN: Vanderbilt University Press.

Edu, Ugo F. 2019. "Aesthetics Politics: Negotiations of Black Reproduction in Brazil." *Medical Anthropology* 38 (8): 680–694.

El Economista. 2015. "Narcotráfico Mexicano Obliga a Doctores a Trabajar en los Territorios que Controlan." *América Economía,* July 1, 2015. https://www.americaeconomia.com/politica -sociedad/politica/narcotrafico-mexicano-obliga-doctores-trabajar-en-los-territorios-que -con.

Enciso, Angélica L. 2014. "Miles de Médicos Demandan no Criminalizar su Actividad." *La Jornada,* June 23, 2014. http://www.jornada.unam.mx/2014/06/23/politica/003n1pol.

Epps Jr., Charles H., Davis G. Johnson, and Audrey L. Vaughan. 1993. "Black Medical Pioneers: African-American 'Firsts' in Academic and Organized Medicine, Part Two." *Journal of the National Medical Association* 85 (9): 703–720.

Excélsior. 2014. "#YoSoy17: La Muerte del Joven que Desató un Movimiento Nacional." *Excélsior,* June 23, 2014. http://www.excelsior.com.mx/nacional/2014/06/23/966856.

Fajardo-Ortiz, Guillermo. 1999. "El Escenario Hospitalario en Puebla durante el Virreinato." *Gaceta Médica de México* 135 (4): 427–431.

———. 2002. "Un Pasado con Mucho Presente: El Hospital Real de San Pedro en Puebla de los Ángeles." *Cirugía y Cirujanos* 70 (6): 459–467.

Falu, Nessette. 2019. "Vivência Negra: Black Lesbians Affective Experiences in Brazilian Gynecology." *Medical Anthropology* 38 (8): 695–709.

Fernández-Ortega, Miguel A., Armando Ortiz-Montalvo, Efrén R. Ponce-Rosas, Guillermo Fajardo-Ortiz, and Juan J. Mazón-Ramírez. 2016. "Caracterización de Alumnos de la Carrera de Medicina." *Investigación en Educación Médica* 5 (19): 148–154.

Files, Julia A., Anita P. Mayer, Marcia G. Ko, Patricia Friedrich, Marjorie Jenkins, Michael J. Bryan, Suneela Vegunta, Christopher M. Wittich, Melissa A. Lyle, and Ryan Melikian. 2017. "Speaker Introductions at Internal Medicine Grand Rounds: Forms of Address Reveal Gender Bias." *Journal of Women's Health* 26 (5): 413–419.

Finkler, Kaja. 2001. *Physicians at Work, Patients in Pain.* Durham, NC: Carolina Academic Press.

———. 2004. "Biomedicine Globalized and Localized: Western Medical Practices in an Outpatient Clinic of a Mexican Hospital." *Social Science and Medicine* 59 (10): 2037–2051.

Foucault, Michel. 1973. *The Birth of the Clinic: An Archaeology of Medical Perception.* Translated by A. M. Sheridan. London: Tavistock.

Frenda, Steven J., and Kimberly M. Fenn. 2016. "Sleep Less, Think Worse: The Effect of Sleep Deprivation on Working Memory." *Journal of Applied Research in Memory and Cognition* 5 (4): 463–469.

Frenk, Julio. 2006. "Bridging the Divide: Global Lessons from Evidence-Based Health Policy in Mexico." *The Lancet* 368 (9539): 954–961.

Frenk, Julio, Octavio Gómez-Dantés, and Felicia Marie Knaul. 2019. "A Dark Day for Universal Health Coverage." *The Lancet* 393 (10169): 301–303.

Frenk, Julio, Eduardo González-Pier, Octavio Gómez-Dantés, Miguel A. Lezana, and Felicia M. Knaul. 2006. "Comprehensive Reform to Improve Health System Performance in Mexico." *The Lancet* 368 (9546): 1524–1534.

Frenk, Julio, Héctor Hernández-Llamas, and Lourdes Alvarez-Klein. 1983. "Análisis Histórico del Internado Rotatorio de Pregrado en México." *Gaceta Médica de México* 119 (2): 87–96.

Galtung, Johan. 1990. "Cultural Violence." *Journal of Peace Research* 27 (3): 291–305.

Gall, Olivia. 2004. "Identidad, Exclusión y Racismo: Reflexiones Teóricas sobre México." *Revista Mexicana de Sociología* 66 (2): 221–259.

Gálvez, Alyshia. 2019. "Transnational Mother Blame: Protecting and Caring in a Globalized Context." *Medical Anthropology* 38 (7): 574–587.

Gamble, Jeanne. 2001. "Modelling the Invisible: The Pedagogy of Craft Apprenticeship." *Studies in Continuing Education* 23 (2): 185–200.

García Procel, Emilio. 2007. "La Compleja Red de Hospitales Mexicanos en el Siglo XX." In *Historia de la Medicina en México,* edited by Carlos Viesca, 271–277. Mexico City: Universidad Nacional Autónoma de México.

Gawande, Atul. 2002. *Complications: A Surgeon's Notes on an Imperfect Science.* New York: Metropolitan Books.

Geertz, Clifford. 1998. "Deep Hanging Out." *New York Review of Books* 45 (16): 69–72.

Gieser, Thorsten. 2008. "Embodiment, Emotion and Empathy: A Phenomenological Approach to Apprenticeship Learning." *Anthropological Theory* 8 (3): 299–318.

Goffman, Ervin. 1959. *The Presentation of Self in Everyday Life.* Garden City, NY: Doubleday Anchor Books.

———. 1961. *Asylums: Essays on the Social Situation of Mental Patients and Other Inmates.* Chicago: Aldine.

Good, Byron J. 1994. *Medicine, Rationality, and Experience.* Cambridge: Cambridge University Press.

Good, Mary-Jo D. 1995a. *American Medicine: The Quest for Competence.* Berkeley: University of California Press.

———. 1995b. "Cultural Studies of Biomedicine: An Agenda for Research." *Social Science and Medicine* 41 (4): 461–473.

———. 2011. "The Inner Life of Medicine: A Commentary on Anthropologies of Clinical Training in the Twenty-First Century." *Culture, Medicine and Psychiatry* 35 (2): 321–327.

Good, Mary-Jo D., and Byron J. Good. 1989. "Disabling Practitioners: Hazards of Learning to Be a Doctor in American Medical Education." *American Journal of Orthopsychiatry* 59 (2): 303–309.

Gottbrath, Laurin-Whitney. 2017. "Mexicans March against Femicide after Teen's Murder." *Al Jazeera,* September 18, 2017. https://www.aljazeera.com/news/2017/09/mexicans-march-femicide-teen-murder-170917234207928.html.

Gowlland, Geoffrey. 2019. "The Sociality of Enskilment." *Ethnos* 84 (3): 508–524.

Gutiérrez-Samperio, César. 2016. "El Movimiento Médico en México (1964–1965). ¿Qué Pasa Medio Siglo Después?" *Gaceta Médica de México* 152: 124–134.

Gutmann, Matthew C. 1996. *The Meanings of Macho: Being a Man in Mexico City.* Berkeley: University of California Press.

———. 2005. "Scoring Men: Vasectomies and the Totemic Illusion of Male Sexuality in Oaxaca." *Culture, Medicine and Psychiatry* 29 (1): 79–101.

Hafferty, Frederic W. 1998. "Beyond Curriculum Reform: Confronting Medicine's Hidden Curriculum." *Academic Medicine* 73 (4): 403–407.

Hafferty, Frederic W., and Ronald Franks. 1994. "The Hidden Curriculum, Ethics Teaching, and the Structure of Medical Education." *Academic Medicine* 69 (11): 861–71.

Haidet, Paul, and Cayla R. Teal. 2015. "Organizing Chaos: A Conceptual Framework for Assessing Hidden Curricula in Medical Education." In *The Hidden Curriculum in Health Professional Education,* edited by Frederic W. Hafferty and Joseph F. O'Donnell, 84–95. Lebanon, NH: Dartmouth College Press.

Han, Sallie. 2013. *Pregnancy in Practice: Expectation and Experience in the Contemporary US.* New York: Berghahn Books.

Haney, Charlotte. 2012. "Imperiled Femininity: The Dismembering of Citizenship in Northern Mexico." *Journal of Latin American and Caribbean Anthropology* 17 (2): 238–256.

Hannig, Anita. 2017. *Beyond Surgery: Injury, Healing, and Religion at an Ethiopian Hospital.* Chicago: University of Chicago Press.

Harris, Anna. 2014. "Encountering the Familiar Unknown: The Hidden Work of Adjusting Medical Practice between Local Settings." *Journal of Contemporary Ethnography* 43 (3): 259–282.

———. 2016. "Listening-Touch, Affect and the Crafting of Medical Bodies through Percussion." *Body and Society* 22 (1): 31–61.

Heinze-Martin, Gerhard, Víctor Hugo Olmedo-Canchola, Germán Bazán-Miranda, Napoléon A. Bernard-Fuentes, and Diana P. Guízar-Sánchez. 2018. "Medical Specialists in Mexico." *Gaceta Médica de México* 154 (3): 342–351.

Henslin, James M., and Mae A. Biggs. 1971. "Dramaturgical Desexualization: The Sociology of the Vaginal Exam." In *Studies in the Sociology of Sex,* edited by James M. Henslin, 243–272. New York: Appleton-Century-Crofts.

Higashi, Robin T., Allison Tillack, Michael A. Steinman, C. Bree Johnston, and G. Michael Harper. 2013. "The 'Worthy' Patient: Rethinking the 'Hidden Curriculum' in Medical Education." *Anthropology and Medicine* 20 (1): 13–23.

Hinojosa, Servando Z. 2002. "'The Hands Know': Bodily Engagement and Medical Impasse in Highland Maya Bonesetting." *Medical Anthropology Quarterly* 16 (1): 22–40.

Hinze, Susan W. 1999. "Gender and the Body of Medicine or at Least Some Body Parts: (Re) Constructing the Prestige Hierarchy of Medical Specialties." *Sociological Quarterly* 40 (2): 217–239.

———. 2004. "'Am I Being Over-Sensitive?' Women's Experience of Sexual Harassment during Medical Training." *Health* 8 (1): 101–127.

Hirschberg, Julia. 1979. "Social Experiment in New Spain: A Prosopographical Study of the Early Settlement at Puebla de los Angeles." *Hispanic American Historical Review* 59 (1): 1–33.

Holmes, Seth M., Angela C. Jenks, and Scott Stonington. 2011. "Clinical Subjectivation: Anthropologies of Contemporary Biomedical Training." *Culture, Medicine, and Psychiatry* 35 (2): 105–112.

Holmes, Seth M., and Maya Ponte. 2011. "En-case-ing the Patient: Disciplining Uncertainty in Medical Student Patient Presentations." *Culture, Medicine, and Psychiatry* 35 (2): 163–182.

Homedes, Núria, and Antonio Ugalde. 2009. "Twenty-Five Years of Convoluted Health Reforms in Mexico." *PLoS Medicine* 6 (8): e1000124.

Howes-Mischel, Rebecca. 2016. "'With This You Can Meet Your Baby': Fetal Personhood and Audible Heartbeats in Oaxacan Public Health." *Medical Anthropology Quarterly* 30 (2): 186–202.

Ingold, Tim. 2000. *The Perception of the Environment: Essays on Livelihood, Dwelling and Skill.* New York: Routledge.

Instituto Nacional Para la Competitividad (IMCO). 2018. Compara Carreras: Medicina. https://imco.org.mx/comparacarreras/carrera/711

Instituto Nacional de Estadística y Geografía (INEGI). 2010. "Cuéntame: Información por Entidad." http://cuentame.inegi.org.mx/monografias/informacion/pue/poblacion/diversidad.aspx?tema=me&e=21.

———. 2014a. "Anuario Estadístico y Geográfico de Puebla 2014." http://internet.contenidos.inegi.org.mx/contenidos/productos/prod_serv/contenidos/espanol/bvinegi/productos/anuario_14/702825066239.pdf

———. 2014b. "Estadísticas a Propósito del Día del Médico (23 De Octubre)." http://www.beta.inegi.org.mx/contenidos/saladeprensa/aproposito/2014/medico0.pdf.

Instituto Nacional de las Mujeres (Inmujeres). 2020. "Alerta de Violencia de Género contra las Mujeres." *Gobierno de México,* January 22, 2020. https://www.gob.mx/inmujeres/acciones-y-programas/alerta-de-violencia-de-genero-contra-las-mujeres-80739.

Instituto de Salud para el Bienestar (INSABI). 2020. "El Gobierno de México avanza en la aplicación de la vacuna contra la COVID-19." https://www.gob.mx/insabi.

Jackson, Michael. 1983. "Knowledge of the Body." *Man* 18 (2): 327–345.

Jaramillo-Tallabs, Sandra E. 2010. "Historias de Vida: La Mujer en la Medicina." *Medicina Universitaria* 12 (46): 70–78.

Jarillo Soto, Edgar C., Manuel O. Lemus, and Addis A. Salinas Urbina. 2011. "Formación y Práctica de Profesionales de la Salud: Una Mirada a su Historia en México." In *La Salud en México,* edited by M. de Consuelo Chapela Mendoza and M. Elena Contrera Garfias, 221–245. Xochimilco: Universidad Autónoma Metropolitana.

Jasso, Carmina, and Karina González. 2018. "Brechas en la Medición de Feminicidios en México." *Resonancias* [UNAM], September 10, 2018. https://www.iis.unam.mx/blog/brechas-en-la-medicion-de-feminicidios-en-mexico/.

Jewkes, Rachel, and Loveday Penn-Kekana. 2015. "Mistreatment of Women in Childbirth: Time for Action on this Important Dimension of Violence against Women." *PLoS Medicine* 12 (6): e1001849.

Jordan, Brigitte. 1997. "Authoritative Knowledge and Its Construction." In *Childbirth and Authoritative Knowledge: Cross-Cultural Perspectives,* edited by Robbie E. Davis-Floyd and Carolyn F. Sargent, 55–79. Berkeley: University of California Press.

Kanitkar, Helen. 1994. "'Real True Boys': Moulding the Cadets of Imperialism." In *Dislocating Masculinity: Comparative Ethnographies,* edited by Andrea Cornwall and Nancy Lindisfarne, 194–196. London: Routledge.

Kay, Jerald. 1990. "Traumatic Deidealization and the Future of Medicine." *Journal of the American Medical Association* (4): 572–573.

Kilshaw, Susie. 2017. "Birds, Meat, and Babies: The Multiple Realities of Fetuses in Qatar." *Anthropology and Medicine* 24 (2): 189–204.

Kitroeff, Natalie, and Paulina Villegas. 2020. "'No Es el Virus': Las Carencias de los Hospitales Mexicanos También Matan." *New York Times,* May 28, 2020. https://www.nytimes.com/es/2020/05/28/espanol/america-latina/mexico-hospitales-coronavirus.html.

Klaber, R. E., and Macdougall, C. F. 2009. "Maximising Learning Opportunities in Handover." *Archives of Disease in Childhood-Education and Practice* 94 (4): 118–122.

Kosambi, Meera. 1996. "Anandibai Joshee: Retrieving a Fragmented Feminist Image." *Economic and Political Weekly* 31 (49): 3189–3197.

Lakhani, Nina. 2015. "Tenancingo: The Small Town at the Dark Heart of Mexico's Sex-Slave Trade." *The Guardian,* April 4, 2015. https://www.theguardian.com/world/2015/apr/05/tenancingo-mexico-sex-slave-trade-america.

Lan, Conrado E. 1995. "Body and Soul in Plato's Anthropology." *Kernos. Revue Internationale et Pluridisciplinaire de Religion Grecque Antique* 8:107–112.

Lave, Jean. 2011. *Apprenticeship in Critical Ethnographic Practice.* Chicago: University of Chicago Press.

Lave, Jean, and Etienne Wenger. 1991. *Situated Learning: Legitimate Peripheral Participation.* Cambridge: Cambridge University Press.

Levi, Primo. (1986) 2017. *The Drowned and the Saved.* Translated from Italian by Raymond Rosenthal. New York: Simon & Schuster Paperbacks.

Livingston, Julie. 2012. *Improvising Medicine: An African Oncology Ward in an Emerging Cancer Epidemic.* Durham, NC: Duke University Press.

Long, Debbi, Cynthia Hunter, and Sjaak van der Geest. 2008. "When the Field Is a Ward or a Clinic: Hospital Ethnography." *Anthropology and Medicine* 15 (2): 71–78.

López-Arellano, Olivia, and José Blanco-Gil. 2001. "La Polarización de la Política de Salud en México." *Cadernos de Saúde Pública, Rio de Janeiro* 17 (1): 43–54.

Luhrmann, Tanya M. 2000. *Of Two Minds: The Growing Disorder in Psychiatry*. New York: Alfred A. Knopf.

———. 2001. "Identity in Anthropology." In *International Encyclopedia of the Social and Behavioral Sciences*, edited by Neil J. Smelser and Paul B. Baltes, 7154–7159. Oxford: Pergamon Press.

Lynn, Christopher D., Michaela E. Howells, and Max J. Stein. 2018. "Family and the Field: Expectations of a Field Based Research Career Affect Researcher's Family Planning Decisions." *PLOS One* 13 (9): e0203500.

Mahtani, Minelle. 2014. "Toxic Geographies: Absences in Critical Race Thought and Practice in Social and Cultural Geography." *Social and Cultural Geography* 15 (4): 359–367.

Malvido, Elsa, and Miguel A. Cuenya Mateos. 2009. "Las Cartillas Médicas y el Cólera Morbus de 1833: El Caso de la Ciudad de Puebla." In *Medicina, Ciencia y Sociedad en México, Siglo XIX*, edited by Laura Cházaro, 125–135. Zamora, México: El Colegio de Michoacán.

Mankaka, Cindy O., Gérard Waeber, and David Gachoud. 2014. "Female Residents Experiencing Medical Errors in General Internal Medicine: A Qualitative Study." *BMC Medical Education* 14 (1): 140.

Martínez Barbosa, Xóchitl. 2007. "Atención y Regulación Médica en los Siglos XVI–XVII." In *Historia de la Medicina en México*, edited by Carlos Viesca, 129–143. Mexico City: Universidad Nacional Autónoma de México.

Martínez Cortés, Fernando. 2007. "La Clínica en México en la Segunda Mitad del Siglo XIX: Antecedentes." In *Historia de la Medicina en México*, edited by Carlos Viesca, 197–219. Mexico City: Universidad Nacional Autónoma de México.

Masood, Ayesha. 2019. "Doing Gender, Modestly: Conceptualizing Workplace Experiences of Pakistani Women Doctors." *Gender, Work and Organization* 26 (2): 214–228.

Matos, Kenneth, Olivia M. O'Neill, and Xue Lei. 2018. "Toxic Leadership and the Masculinity Contest Culture: How 'Win or Die' Cultures Breed Abusive Leadership." *Journal of Social Issues* 74 (3): 500–528.

Mauss, Marcel. 1973. "Techniques of the Body." *Economy and Society* 2:70–88.

Mbembé, Achille. 2003. "Necropolitics." *Public Culture* 15 (1): 11–40.

McElhinny, Bonnie. 1994. "An Economy of Affect: Objectivity, Masculinity and the Gendering of Police Work." In *Dislocating Masculinity*, edited by Andrea Cornwall and Nancy Lindisfarne, 159–171. London: Routledge.

Mendoza Escamilla, Viridiana. 2019. "México, Sin Dinero para un Sistema de Salud Universal." *Forbes México*, June 12, 2019. https://www.forbes.com.mx/foro-forbes-salud-2019-mexico-sin-dinero-para-un-sistema-de-salud-universal/#:~:text=La%20investigadora%20explica%20que%20el,como%20la%20seguridad%20osocial%20p%C3%BAblica.

Mirandé, Alfredo. 2018. *Hombres y Machos: Masculinity and Latino Culture*. New York: Routledge.

Mol, Annmarie. 2003. *The Body Multiple: Ontology in Medical Practice*. Durham, NC: Duke University Press.

Molyneux, Maxine. 2000. "Twentieth-Century State Formations in Latin America." In *Hidden Histories of Gender and the State in Latin America*, edited by Elizabeth Dore and Maxine Molyneux, 33–81. Durham, NC: Duke University Press.

Montes-Villaseñor, Evangelina, Janet García-González, María S. L. Blázquez-Morales, Alma Cruz-Juárez, and Xóchitl M. De-San-Jorge-Cárdenas. 2018. "Exposición a la Violencia Durante la Formación Profesional de los Residentes Médicos." *CienciaUAT* 12 (2): 54–66.

Monteverde, Eduardo, and Gabino Sánchez. 2007. "Tradición e Innovación en la Enseñanza de la Medicina de la Colonia a la Nación (1820–1850)." In *Historia de la Medicina en México*, edited by Carlos Viesca, 187–195. Mexico City: Universidad Nacional Autónoma de México.

Morales, Gabriela E. 2018. "There Is No Place Like Home: Imitation and the Politics of Recognition in Bolivian Obstetric Care." *Medical Anthropology Quarterly* 32 (3), 404–424.

Morales-Gómez, Antonio, and Alda M. Medina-Figueroa. 2007. "Percepción del Alumno de Pregrado de Medicina, Acerca del Ambiente Educativo en el IMSS." *Revista Médica del Instituto Mexicano del Seguro Social* 45 (2): 123–131.

Nader, Laura. 1972. "Up the Anthropologist: Perspectives Gained from Studying Up." In *Reinventing Anthropology*, edited by Dell Hymes, 284–311. New York: Vintage Books.

Nájar, Alberto. 2017. "Feminicidio en México: Mara Castilla, el Asesinato de una Joven de 19 Años en un Taxi que Indigna a un País Violento." *BBC News: Mundo*, September 18, 2017. https://www.bbc.com/mundo/noticias-america-latina-41303542.

Nigenda, Gustavo, and Armando Solórzano. 1997. "Doctors and Corporatist Politics: The Case of the Mexican Medical Profession." *Journal of Health Politics, Policy, and Law* 22 (1): 73–99.

Nutini, Hugo G. 1997. "Class and Ethnicity in Mexico: Somatic and Racial Considerations." *Ethnology* 36 (3): 227–238.

Oboler, Suzanne, and Anani Dzidzienyo. 2005. "Flows and Counterflows: Latinas/os, Blackness, and Racialization in Hemispheric Perspective." In *Neither Enemies nor Friends: Latinos, Blacks, and Afro-Latinos*, edited by Anani Dzidzienyo and Suzanne Oboler, 3–35. New York: Palgrave Macmillan.

O'Brien, Elizabeth. 2013. "Pelvimetry and the Persistence of Racial Science in Obstetrics." *Endeavour* 37 (1): 21–28.

O'Connor, Anne-Marie, and William Booth. 2010. "Mexico's Medical Workers on the Front Lines of Drug War." *Washington Post*, November 19, 2010. http://www.washingtonpost.com/wp-dyn/content/article/2010/11/18/AR2010111806395.html.

O'Donnell, Joseph. 2015. "Introduction: The Hidden Curriculum—a Focus on Learning and Closing the Gap." In *The Hidden Curriculum in Health Professional Education*, edited by Frederic W. Hafferty and Joseph F. O'Donnell, 1–20. Lebanon, NH: Dartmouth College Press.

Olvera, Dulce. 2019. "Depresión, Peleas a Golpazos, y Suicidios en los Hospitales Mexicanos por el Acoso y Violencia Contra Médicos." *Telemundo*, November 18, 2019. https://www.telemundo.com/noticias/2019/11/18/depresion-peleas-golpazos-y-suicidios-en-los-hospitales-mexicanos-por-el-acoso-y-violencia-tmna3585548.

Organisation for Economic Co-operation and Development (OECD). 2020. "Health Resources: Doctors." https://doi.org/10.1787/777a9575-en.

Ortiz-Acosta, R., and B. E. Beltrán-Jiménez. 2011. "Inteligencia Emocional Percibida y Desgaste Laboral en Médicos Internos de Pregrado." *Educación Médica* 14 (1): 49–55.

Ortner, Sherry B. 1974. "Is Female to Male as Nature Is to Culture?" In *Woman, Culture, and Society*, edited by Michelle Z. Rosaldo and Louise Lamphere, 68–87. Stanford, CA: Stanford University Press.

Padilla, Lizbeth. 2018. "La Inseguridad Pega a la Salud: Médicos Abandonan Centros de Salud de la Sierra de Chihuahua." *Animal Político*, August 18, 2018. https://www.animalpolitico.com/2018/08/la-inseguridad-pega-a-la-salud-medicos-abandonan-centros-de-salud-de-la-sierra-de-chihuahua/.

Paice, Elisabeth, Shelley Heard, and Fiona Moss. 2002. "How Important Are Role Models in Making Good Doctors?" *British Medical Journal* 325 (7366): 707–710.

Pálsson, Gísli. 1994. "Enskilment at Sea." *Man* 29 (4): 901–927.

Pensado, Jaime M. 2013. *Rebel Mexico: Student Unrest and Authoritarian Political Culture during the Long Sixties*. Stanford, CA: Stanford University Press.

Pérez Oseguera, María de L., and Anahí Espíndola Pérez. 2015. *Mujeres Desaparecidas en Puebla: Informe 2005–2009*. Puebla, México: Universidad Iberoamericana Puebla.

Perlman, Nicola C., and Daniela A. Carusi. 2019. "Retained Placenta after Vaginal Delivery: Risk Factors and Management." *International Journal of Women's Health* 11:527–532.

Piemonte, Nicole M. 2015. "Last Laughs: Gallows Humor and Medical Education." *Journal of Medical Humanities* 36 (4): 375–380.

Pink, Sarah, Jennie Morgan, and Andrew Dainty. 2014. "The Safe Hand: Gels, Water, Gloves and the Materiality of Tactile Knowing." *Journal of Material Culture* 19 (4): 425–442.

Pollock, Donald. 1996. "Training Tales: US Medical Autobiography." *Cultural Anthropology* 11 (3): 339–361.

Pozas Horcasitas, Ricardo. 1993. *La Democracia en Blanco: El Movimiento Médico en México, 1964–1965*. Mexico City: Siglo XXI Editores.

Prentice, Rachel. 2005. "The Anatomy of a Surgical Simulation: The Mutual Articulation of Bodies in and through the Machine." *Social Studies of Science* 35 (6): 837–866.

———. 2013. *Bodies in Formation: An Ethnography of Anatomy and Surgery Education*. Durham, NC: Duke University Press.

Programa de las Naciones Unidas para el Desarrollo (PNUD). 2014. *El Desarrollo Humano y los Objetivos de Desarrollo del Milenio en Puebla*. New York: Programa de las Naciones Unidas para el Desarrollo.

Rabow, Michael W. 2015. "Becoming a Doctor: Learning from the Hidden Curriculum in Medical Education." In *The Hidden Curriculum in Health Professional Education*, edited by Frederic W. Hafferty and Joseph F. O'Donnell, 130–139. Lebanon, NH: Dartmouth College Press.

Radio Fórmula. 2014. "Defiende SNTSS a Médicos Acusados de Supuesta Negligencia Médica." *Radio Fórmula*, June 12, 2014. http://www.radioformula.com.mx/notas.asp?Idn=418376&idFC=2014.

Ramírez, Paul. 2012. "'Like Herod's Massacre': Quarantines, Bourbon Reform, and Popular Protest in Oaxaca's Smallpox Epidemic, 1796–1797." *The Americas* 69 (2): 203–235.

Ramírez-Ortega, Verónica. 2010. "La Enseñanza de las Profesiones Médica y Quirúrgica Hacia el Final del Régimen Colonial." *Revista Médica del Instituto Mexicano del Seguro Social* 48 (2): 159–162.

Ramos, Frances L. 2012. *Identity, Ritual, and Power in Colonial Puebla*. Tucson: University of Arizona Press.

Rapp, Rayna. 2019. "Race and Reproduction: An Enduring Conversation." *Medical Anthropology* 38(8): 725–732.

Rello, Maricarmen. 2014. "Ordenan Aprehender a 16 Médicos del IMSS por Negligencia en Jalisco." *Milenio*, June 4, 2014. http://www.milenio.com/region/Liberan-ordenes-aprehension-IMSS-Jalisco_0_311369079.html.

Reuters. 2020. "México Supera a EU y Brasil en Muertes de Personal Médico por COVID-19." *Alto Nivel*, June 8, 2020. https://www.altonivel.com.mx/actualidad/mexico-supera-a-eu-y-brasil-en-muertes-de-personal-medico-por-covid-19/.

Reyes Carmona, Carlos, Ana M. Monterrosas Rojas, Andrea Navarrete Martínez, Estephanie P. Acosta Martínez, and Uri Torruco García. 2017. "Ansiedad de los Estudiantes de una Facultad de Medicina Mexicana, Antes de Iniciar el Internado." *Investigación en Educación Médica* 6 (21): 42–46.

Reyes-Foster, Beatriz M. 2016. "Latour's AIME, Indigenous Critique, and Ontological Turns in a Mexican Psychiatric Hospital: Approaching Registers of Visibility in Three Conceptual Turns." *Anthropological Quarterly* 89 (4): 1175–1200.

———. 2018. *Psychiatric Encounters: Madness and Modernity in Yucatan, Mexico*. New Brunswick, NJ: Rutgers University Press.

Rice, Tom. 2010. "'The Hallmark of a Doctor': The Stethoscope and the Making of Medical Identity." *Journal of Material Culture* 15 (3): 287–301.

Riquer Fernández, Florinda, and Roberto Castro. 2012. *Estudio Nacional sobre las Fuentes, Orígenes y Factores que Producen y Reproducen la Violencia contra las Mujeres.* Mexico City: CONAVIM-Centro Regional de Investigaciones Multidisciplinarias UNAM.

Riska, Elianne, and Aurelija Novelskaite. 2008. "Gendered Careers in Post-Soviet Society: Views on Professional Qualifications in Surgery and Pediatrics." *Gender Issues* 25 (4): 229–245.

Roberts, Dorothy. 1997. *Killing the Black Body: Race, Reproduction and the Meaning of Liberty.* New York: Pantheon.

Roberts, Elizabeth F. 2012. "Scars of Nation: Surgical Penetration and the Ecuadorian State." *Journal of Latin American and Caribbean Anthropology* 17 (2): 215–237.

———. 2016. "Gods, Germs, and Petri Dishes: Toward a Nonsecular Medical Anthropology." *Medical Anthropology* 35 (3): 209–219.

Robles Galindo, Rosario. 2012. *En Puebla: Médicos, Ciencia y Academia (1850–1910), El Estudio de la Clínica-Hospitalaria.* Puebla, México: Benemérita Universidad Autónoma de Puebla.

Rodríguez, Martha E. 2007. "La Medicina Novohispana en el Period Ilustrado." In *Historia de la Medicina en México,* edited by Carlos Viesca, 151–163. Mexico City: Universidad Nacional Autónoma de México.

———. 2008. *La Escuela Nacional de Medicina 1833–1910. Monografías de Historia y Filosofía de la Medicina, Num. 5.* Mexico City: Universidad Nacional Autónoma de México.

———. 2010. "La Escuela Nacional de Medicina en los Tiempos del Centenario." *Revista Médica del Instituto Mexicano del Seguro Social* 48 (4): 405–414.

Rodríguez de Romo, Ana C., and Martha E. Rodríguez Pérez. 1998. "Historia de la Salud Pública en México: Siglos XIX y XX." *História, Ciências, Saúde—Manguinhos* 5 (2): 293–310.

Rodríguez-Sala, María L. 2005. *Los Cirujanos de Hospitales de la Nueva España (Siglos XVI y XVII): ¿Miembros de un Estamento Profesional o de una Comunidad Científica?* Mexico City: Universidad Nacional Autónoma de México.

Rojas, Clara E. 2005. "The 'V-Day' March in Mexico: Appropriation and Misuse of Local Women's Activism." *NWSA Journal* 17 (2): 217–227.

Romero-Huesca, Andrés, and Julio Ramírez-Bollas. 2003. "La Atención Médica en el Hospital Real de Naturales." *Cirugía y Cirujanos* 71 (6): 496–503.

Rose, Mike. 1999. "'Our Hands Will Know': The Development of Tactile Diagnostic Skill— Teaching, Learning, and Situated Cognition in a Physical Therapy Program." *Anthropology and Education Quarterly* 30 (2): 133–160.

Rouse, Joseph. 2013. "What Is Conceptually Articulated Understanding?" In *Mind, Reason, and Being-in-the-Word,* edited by Joseph K. Schear, 250–271. London: Routledge.

Rubin, Sarah. 2015. "Everyday Acts of Violence and Resistance: Motherhood and Childbirth in the South African Township Maternity Clinic." Paper presented the 114th Annual Meeting of the American Anthropological Association, Denver, CO, November 2015.

Ruiz, Apen. 2001. "La India Bonita: Nación, Raza y Género en el México Revolucionario." *Debate Feminista* 24:142–162.

Sadler, Michelle, Mário J. D. S. Santos, Dolores Ruiz-Berdún, Gonzalo Leiva Rojas, Elena Skoko, Patricia Gillen, and Jette A. Clausen. 2016. "Moving beyond Disrespect and Abuse: Addressing the Structural Dimensions of Obstetric Violence." *Reproductive Health Matters* 24 (47): 47–55.

Saldaña-Tejeda, Abril, and Peter Wade. 2019. "Eugenics, Epigenetics, and Obesity Predisposition among Mexican Mestizos." *Medical Anthropology* 38(8): 664–679.

Salhi, Bisan. 2016. "Beyond the Doctor's White Coat: Science, Ritual, and Healing in American Biomedicine." In *Understanding and Applying Medical Anthropology: Biosocial and Cultural Approaches,* edited by Peter J. Brown and Svea Closser, 204–212. New York: Routledge.

Sanfilippo, José B. 2007. "El Surgimiento de la Medcina Mexicana: Aculturación y Resignifi-cación." In *Historia de la Medicina en México*, edited by Carlos Viesca, 113–127. Mexico City: Universidad Nacional Autónoma de México.

Sánchez Hernández, Andrés A., and Gracia Dorel-Ferré. 2008. *Casa de Maternidad: Fundación Luis de Haro y Tamariz*. Puebla, México: Benemérita Universidad Autónoma de Puebla.

Santana, Rosa. 2013. "Claman Justicia por Asesinato de Médico Pasante en Campeche." *Proceso*, November 28, 2013. https://www.proceso.com.mx/359140/claman-justicia-por-asesinato -de-medico-pasante-en-campeche.

Saul, Heather. 2015. "Exhausted Doctors Post Pictures of Themselves Asleep at Work to High-light How Tiring Shifts Are." *Independent*, May 19, 2015. https://www.independent.co.uk /news/world/americas/exhausted-doctors-post-pictures-of-themselves-asleep-at-work -to-highlight-how-tiring-shifts-are-10259969.html.

Savage, Virginia, and Arachu Castro. 2017. "Measuring Mistreatment of Women during Child-birth: A Review of Terminology and Methodological Approaches." *Reproductive Health* 14 (1): 138.

Scheper-Hughes, Nancy, and Margaret M. Lock. 1987. "The Mindful Body: A Prolegomenon to Future Work in Medical Anthropology." *Medical Anthropology Quarterly*, New Series 1 (1): 6–41

Secretaría de Salud. 2016. *Informe Sobre la Salud de los Mexicanos 2016: Diagnóstico General del Sistema Nacional de Salud*. Mexico City: Secretaría de Salud. https://www.gob.mx/cms /uploads/attachment/file/239410/ISSM_2016.pdf.

———. 2017. "Salubridad Pública: Procedencia Institucional." Archivo Histórico de la Secre-taría de Salud. https://web.archive.org/web/20180809043131/http://pliopencms05.salud .gob.mx:8080/archivo/ahssa/salubridad.

Setola, Nicoletta, Sabrina Borgianni, Max Martinez, and Eime Tobari. 2013. "The Role of Spatial Layout of Hospital Public Spaces in Informal Patient-Medical Staff Interface." In *Proceed-ings of the Ninth International Space Syntax Symposium*, edited by Y. O. Kim, H. T. Park, and K. W. Seo, 025. Seoul: Sejong University. http://sss9sejong.or.kr/paperpdf/bmp/SSS9 _2013_REF025_P.pdf.

Sharp, Lesley A. 2000. "The Commodification of the Body and Its Parts." *Annual Review of Anthropology* 29:287–328.

Sherman, Christopher. 2020. "Médicos en México Denuncian Falta de Equipo y Capacit-ación." *Chicago Tribune*, April 13, 2020. https://www.chicagotribune.com/espanol/sns-es -coronavirus-medicos-denuncian-falta-equipo-en-mexico-20200413-7hfattfelffutgqkc3v6s- s7urm-story.html.

Shetty, Jyothi, Vinod Aahir, Deeksha Pandey, Prashanth Adiga, and Asha Kamath. 2014. "Fetal Head Position during the First Stage of Labor: Comparison between Vaginal Exam-ination and Transabdominal Ultrasound." *ISRN Obstetrics and Gynecology* 2014:314617.

Sieler, Roman. 2014. "Patient Agency Revisited: 'Healing the Hidden' in South India." *Medical Anthropology Quarterly* 28 (3): 323–341.

Singer, Elyse O. 2017. "From Reproductive Rights to Responsibilization: Fashioning Liberal Subjects in Mexico City's New Public Sector Abortion Program." *Medical Anthropology Quarterly* 31 (4): 445–463.

Smith-Oka, Vania. 2013a. "Managing Labor and Delivery among Impoverished Populations in Mexico: Cervical Examinations as Bureaucratic Practice." *American Anthropologist* 115 (4): 595–607.

———. 2013b. *Shaping the Motherhood of Indigenous Mexico*. Nashville, TN: Vanderbilt Uni-versity Press.

———. 2015. "Microaggressions and the Reproduction of Social Inequalities in Medical Encounters in Mexico." *Social Science and Medicine* 143:9–16.

Smith-Oka, Vania, and Megan K. Marshalla. 2019. "Crossing Bodily, Social, and Intimate Boundaries: How Class, Ethnic, and Gender Differences Are Reproduced in Medical Training in Mexico." *American Anthropologist* 121 (1): 113–125.

Sosa-Rubí, Sandra G., Aarón Salinas-Rodríguez, and Omar Galárraga. 2011. "Impacto del Seguro Popular en el Gasto Catastrófico y de Bolsillo en el México Rural y Urbano, 2005–2008." *Salud Pública de México* 53 (S4): 425–435.

Soto Laveaga, Gabriela. 2013a. "Shadowing the Professional Class: Reporting Fictions in Doctors' Strikes." *Journal of Iberian and Latin American Research* 19 (1): 30–40.

———. 2013b. "Seeing the Countryside through Medical Eyes: Social Service Reports in the Making of a Sickly Nation." *Endeavour* 37 (1): 29–38.

———. 2013c. "Bringing the Revolution to Medical Schools: Social Service and a Rural Health Emphasis in 1930s Mexico." *Mexican Studies/Estudios Mexicanos* 29 (2): 397–427.

———. 2015. "Building the Nation of the Future, One Waiting Room at a Time: Hospital Murals in the Making of Modern Mexico." *History and Technology* 31 (3): 275–294.

Soto Laveaga, Gabriela, and Claudia Agostoni. 2011. "Science and Public Health in the Century of Revolution." In *A Companion to Mexican History and Culture,* edited by William H. Beezley, 561–574. Hoboken, NJ: Wiley-Blackwell.

Soto-Vega, Elena, Marta Urrutia-Osorio, Fernando Arellano-Valdez, Yazmin I. López-Begines, and Christian H. Hernández-Romero. 2015. "The Epidemic of the Cesarean Section in Private Hospital in Puebla, México." *Obstetrics and Gynecology International Journal* 2 (6): 00058.

Stern, Alexandra M. 1999. "Mestizophilia, Biotypology, and Eugenics in Post-Revolutionary Mexico: Towards a History of Science and the State, 1920–1960." Working Papers Series. Chicago: Mexican Studies Program, Center for Latin American Studies.

Stern, David T. 2015. "A Hidden Narrative." In *The Hidden Curriculum in Health Professional Education,* edited by Frederic W. Hafferty and Joseph F. O'Donnell, 23–31. Lebanon, NH: Dartmouth College Press.

Stonington, Scott D. 2012. "On Ethical Locations: The Good Death in Thailand, Where Ethics Sit in Places." *Social Science and Medicine* 75 (5): 836–844.

Street, Alice. 2014. *Biomedicine in an Unstable Place: Infrastructure and Personhood in a Papua New Guinean Hospital.* Durham, NC: Duke University Press.

Street, Alice, and Simon Coleman. 2012. "Introduction: Real and Imagined Spaces." *Space and Culture* 15 (1): 4–17.

Taylor, Janelle S., and Claire Wendland. 2015. "The Hidden Curriculum in Medicine's 'Culture of No Culture.'" In *The Hidden Curriculum in Health Professional Education,* edited by Frederic W. Hafferty and Joseph F. O'Donnell, 53–62. Lebanon, NH: Dartmouth College Press.

Telles, Edward, René D. Flores, and Fernando Urrea-Giraldo. 2015. "Pigmentocracies: Educational Inequality, Skin Color and Census Ethnoracial Identification in Eight Latin American Countries." *Research in Social Stratification and Mobility* 40:39–58.

Teman, Elly. 2010. *Birthing a Mother: The Surrogate Body and the Pregnant Self.* Berkeley: University of California Press.

Turner, Trudy R., Robin M. Bernstein, and Andrea B. Taylor. 2018. "Participation, Representation, and Shared Experiences of Women Scholars in Biological Anthropology." *American Journal of Physical Anthropology* 165 (S65): 126–157.

Turner, Victor. 1967. *The Forest of Symbols: Aspects of Ndembu Ritual.* Ithaca, NY: Cornell University Press.

Tweedy, Damon. 2015. *Black Man in a White Coat: A Doctor's Reflections on Race and Medicine.* New York: Picador.

UN Women. 2017. "The Long Road to Justice, Prosecuting Femicide in Mexico." http://www .unwomen.org/en/news/stories/2017/11/feature-prosecuting-femicide-in-mexico.

Ureste, Manu. 2016a. "YoSoyMédico17 Convoca otra Marcha Nacional el 23 de Octubre, Tras Recorte a Salud." *Animal Político,* September 15, 2016. http://www.animalpolitico.com /2016/09/medicos-demandas-marcha-23-octubre/.

———. 2016b. "Lo Mejor de Animal Político en 2016: Hospitales Llenos y sin Medicinas, el Calvario de Pacientes." *Animal Político*, September 15, 2016. https://www.animalpolitico .com/2016/12/hospitales-saturados-y-sin-medicinas-el-calvario-de-pacientes-y-doctores/.

Urner, Fiona, Roland Zimmermann, and Alexander Krafft. 2014. "Manual Removal of the Placenta after Vaginal Delivery: An Unsolved Problem in Obstetrics." *Journal of Pregnancy* 2014: 274651.

Valdez, Natali, and Daisy Deomampo. 2019. "Centering Race and Racism in Reproduction." *Medical Anthropology* 38 (7): 551–559.

Valdez-Santiago, Rosario, Elisa Hidalgo-Solórzano, Mariana Mojarro-Iñiguez, and Luz M. Arenas-Monreal. 2013. "Nueva Evidencia a un Viejo Problema: El Abuso de las Mujeres en las Salas de Parto." *Revista CONAMED* 18 (1): 14–20.

Van der Geest, Sjaak, and Kaja Finkler. 2004. "Hospital Ethnography: Introduction." *Social Science and Medicine* 59 (10): 1995–2001.

Van der Sijpt, Erica. 2018. "The Pain and Pride of 'Angel Mothers': Disappointments and Desires around Reproductive Loss in Romania." *Medical Anthropology* 37 (2): 174–187.

Van Dongen, Els, and Riekje Elema. 2001. "The Art of Touching: The Culture of 'Body Work' in Nursing." *Anthropology and Medicine* 8 (2–3): 149–162.

Van Drie, Melissa. 2013. "Training the Ausculative Ear: Medical Textbooks and Teaching Tapes (1950–2010)." *Senses and Society* 8 (2): 165–191.

Van Gennep, Arnold. 2010. *The Rites of Passage.* Chicago: University of Chicago Press.

Vargas-Bustamante, Arturo, and Claudio A. Méndez. 2014. "Health Care Privatization in Latin America: Comparing Divergent Privatization Approaches in Chile, Colombia, and Mexico." *Journal of Health Politics, Policy, and Law* 39 (4): 841–886.

Vaughan, Mary Kay. 2000. "Modernizing Patriarchy: State Policies, Rural Households, and Women in Mexico, 1930–1940." In *Hidden Histories of Gender and the State in Latin America,* edited by Elizabeth Dore and Maxine Molyneux, 194–214. Durham, NC: Duke University Press.

Vega, Rosalynn A. 2018. *No Alternative: Childbirth, Citizenship, and Indigenous Culture in Mexico.* Austin: University of Texas Press.

Velazco, Alejandro. 2014. "'No Hay Errores, Son Sobrecargas de Trabajo,' Afirman Médicos Mexicanos." *Vice,* June 27, 2014. https://www.vice.com/es_mx/article/gq7pe3/no-hay -errores-son-sobrecargas-de-trabajo-afirman-medicos-mexicanos.

Villalpando, Rubén, and Miroslava Breach. 2010. "Médicos de Ciudad Juárez Paran Labores para Exigir se Frene la Ola de Violencia." *La Jornada,* December 14, 2010. https://www .jornada.com.mx/2010/12/14/politica/013n1pol.

Watson, Katie. 2011. "Gallows Humor in Medicine." *Hastings Center Report* 41 (5): 37–45.

Watson, Timothy, Eduard Shantsila, and Gregory YH Lip. 2009. "Mechanisms of Thrombogenesis in Atrial Fibrillation: Virchow's Triad Revisited." *The Lancet* 373 (9658): 155–166.

Wear, Delese, Joe Zarconi, and Rebecca Garden. 2015. "Disorderly Conduct: Calling Out the Hidden Curriculum(s) of Professionalism." In *The Hidden Curriculum in Health Professional Education,* edited by Frederic W. Hafferty and Joseph F. O'Donnell, 63–72. Lebanon, NH: Dartmouth College Press.

Wendland, Claire L. 2007. "The Vanishing Mother: Cesarean Section and 'Evidence-Based Obstetrics.'" *Medical Anthropology Quarterly* 21 (2): 218–233.

———. 2010. *A Heart for the Work: Journeys through an African Medical School.* Chicago: University of Chicago Press.

Wentzell, Emily A. 2013. *Maturing Masculinities: Aging, Chronic Illness, and Viagra in Mexico.* Durham, NC: Duke University Press.

Werman, Marco, and Christopher Woolf. 2013. "Historical Photos Depict Women Medical Pioneers." *Public Radio International,* July 12, 2013. https://www.pri.org/stories/2013-07-12/historical-photos-depict-women-medical-pioneers.

Williamson, K. Eliza. 2019. Roundtable panelist in "Responding to the Problem of Violence, Disrespect and Abuse within Maternal Healthcare." Presented at the Joint Meeting of the American Anthropological Association/Canadian Anthropology Society, Vancouver, BC, Canada, November 2019.

World Health Organization (WHO). 2015. "The Prevention and Elimination of Disrespect and Abuse during Facility-Based Childbirth." http://apps.who.int/iris/bitstream/10665/134588/1/WHO_RHR_14.23_eng.pdf.

———. 2018a. "WHO Recommendation on Digital Vaginal Examination." https://extranet.who.int/rhl/topics/preconception-pregnancy-childbirth-and-postpartum-care/care-during-childbirth/care-during-labour-1st-stage/who-recommendation-digital-vaginal-examination.

———. 2018b. "WHO Recommendation on Fundal Pressure to Facilitate Childbirth." https://extranet.who.int/rhl/topics/preconception-pregnancy-childbirth-and-postpartum-care/care-during-childbirth/care-during-labour-2nd-stage/who-recommendation-fundal-pressure-facilitate-childbirth.

———. 2019. "Density of Physicians (Total Number Per 1000 Population, Latest Available Year)." https://www.who.int/gho/health_workforce/physicians_density/en/.

Wright, Melissa W. 2011. "Necropolitics, Narcopolitics, and Femicide: Gendered Violence on the Mexico-US Border." *Signs: Journal of Women in Culture and Society* 36 (3): 707–731.

Young, Katharine G. 1997. *Presence in the Flesh: The Body in Medicine.* Cambridge, MA: Harvard University Press.

Zaman, Shahaduz. 2005. *Broken Limbs, Broken Lives: Ethnography of a Hospital Ward in Bangladesh.* Amsterdam: Het Spinhuis.

Žižek, Slavoj. 2008. *Violence: Six Sideways Reflections.* New York: Picador.

INDEX

Note: Page numbers in *italics* refer to illustrative matter.

ABOUT THE AUTHOR

VANIA SMITH-OKA is an associate professor in the Department of Anthropology at the University of Notre Dame. A sociocultural and medical anthropologist, she has published widely on reproduction, hospital ethnography, development, motherhood, risk, and obstetric violence, including her first book, *Shaping the Motherhood of Indigenous Mexico* (2013).

Available titles in the Medical Anthropology:
Health, Inequality, and Social Justice series